Becoming a Doctor: Is Really the Career for You?

Edited by
Tom Nolan and Matt Green

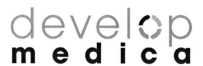

Published by Developmedica
Castle Court
Duke Street
New Basford
Nottingham, NG7 7JN
0845 8380571
www.developmedica.com

Developmedica recommend that you consult the Universities and Colleges Admissions Service (UCAS) and medical school websites for information relating to guidance on how to apply to a university in the UK. Developmedica are neither endorsed by or affiliated with any medical schools or UCAS.

The contents of this book are intended as a guide only and although every effort has been made to ensure that the contents of this book are correct, Developmedica cannot be held responsible for the outcome of any loss or damage that arises through the use of this guide. Readers are advised to seek independent advice regarding their medical school application together with consulting institutions the reader intends to apply to.

A catalogue record for this title is available from the British Library

ISBN 978–0–9556746–6–2

Typeset by RefineCatch Limited, Bungay, Suffolk
Printed by Bell and Bain, Glasgow

1 2 3 4 5 6 7 8 9 10

Contents

Chapter 3:   What steps are involved in the application process?

Gayathri Rabindra

Chapter 4:   How to choose which medical school to apply for

Matthew Harrison

Chapter 5:   What is life like as a medical student?   33
Matthew Harrison

Chapter 6: Mature or graduate entry medicine – what is it all about? 45

Catherine Cheesman

Chapter 7: Student finances **57**
Dina Mansour

The costs 58
Funding your application 58
Tuition fees 59
Living costs 59
In-course costs 61
Student memberships 61
Elective 62
Estimating your income 62
Student loan 62
Grants and bursaries 62
Bank loans 63
Other sources of funding 63
Summary 65

Chapter 8: What do the early years of medical school involve? **67**
Matthew Harrison

Teaching methods 70
Exams 73
Intercalation 75
What sort of things can you study? 75
To intercalate, or not to intercalate? 75

Chapter 9: Reaching your goal 79
Tom Nolan

Chapter 10:   Career paths **93**
Tom Nolan

Chapter 11: What is it like to be a physician?

Amit Bali

Chapter 12: Life as a Surgeon – What is all the hype?

Chris Thompson

Chapter 13: Psychiatry – what's it all about?

Jamie Wilson

About the Editors

Tom Nolan, MBBS BSc

Tom Nolan graduated from the Royal Free and University College Medical School in 2006. He worked as a junior doctor in the London area, where he completed his foundation training. He currently works at the British Medical Journal as a Clinical Editor. He has been a facilitator on the Developmedica Medical School Interview Workshops since 2007.

Matt Green, BSc MPhil

After establishing a private tuition service in 2004, Matt went on to found Developmedica in 2005, and for the last five years has been supporting prospective medical and dental students secure their first choice university place.

List of Contributors

Gayathri Rabindra, MBBS MA (Cantab) Gayathri Rabindra studied pre-clinical medicine at Cambridge University and completed her medical degree at Royal Free and University College Medical School. She is currently a GP ST1 on the Sidcup Vocational Training Scheme, having successfully gained a place in the London Deanery. She is also involved in the GPST courses for Developmedica.

Matt Harrison is a fourth year medical student at the University of Nottingham with an interest in mental health and respiratory medicine.

Catherine Cheesman BMedSci MCSP MSC (Erg) is a fourth year medical student at the University of Nottingham. She trained as a physiotherapist and did her Masters degree in ergonomics and prevention of work related injury before applying to medicine.

Dina Mansour MBBS MA (Cantab) completed her pre-clinical studies at Cambridge University and transferred to Royal Free and University College medical school for clinical training. She now works as a core medical trainee in Brighton and Sussex University Hospital Trust as a core medical trainee.

Amit Bali MBBS BSc is currently training as an ST1 in Paediatrics in East London. He has previously worked in

General Medicine, including Chest Medicine, Diabetes and Endocrinology, Oncology and Emergency Medicine.

Chris Thompson MBChB MRCS (Ed) is a third year general surgery trainee in the West Midlands.

Jamie Wilson MBChB MRCPsych qualified in medicine from Leeds University Medical School. He is a member of the Royal College of Psychiatrists and a former editor at the British Medical Journal Publishing Group.

Chapter 1 Introduction

Doctors are the most trusted members of society. People tell doctors their most intimate thoughts and worries in the hope that they will make them feel better. Doctors are called upon at the most difficult times in peoples' lives – in times of pain, anguish and despair. They offer hope and comfort during these times because of their knowledge, experience and ability to communicate. This privileged position comes at a price: television programmes, for example, paint doctors as hard-working, attractive, intelligent, knowledgeable, caring, decisive and so on. The public expect these things of their doctors and they can be almost impossible to live up to (looking attractive at the end of a 12 hour night shift is particularly tough). However, this is the deal that doctors make with society: in exchange for their unique status, a well paid job and the privilege of being allowed into people's lives they must commit themselves to striving towards giving the best possible care for their patients. This commitment must be shown throughout their careers and must begin several years before becoming a doctor when applying to medical school. It is no wonder then that many people who consider medicine as a career find it a difficult decision to make. Fortunately, help is at hand.

This book aims to help anyone who is considering a career in medicine to make a decision based on all the facts. It begins by asking the biggest question of all: is medicine the career for you? As the chapter explains, doctors come in all shapes and sizes. Some doctors love hammering nails into bones, some enjoy looking at cells under a microscope, and others find helping people cope with incurable illnesses very rewarding. You don't have to want to do all three to have a fulfilling career in medicine. However, there are certain attributes that are likely to make you a good doctor and, just as importantly, make you likely to enjoy this career. Medical schools have a clear idea of the type of people that they are looking for. They have a big responsibility as the large majority of the candidates that they accept will go on to become doctors. As a result, the application process is tough and only the best candidates get offered places. Medical schools are open about the type of students that they want, so if you go about it the right way, there's no reason why your application shouldn't stand out from the rest. With the right preparation you can dramatically improve your chances of being offered a place.

As well as thinking about whether you've got what it takes to be a doctor, you should also ask yourself another question: has medicine got what it takes to satisfy you? Many people have a strange idea of what the day-to-day job of a doctor really involves. One misconception, that you might be relieved is not true, is that as soon as you qualify you are performing operations alone or having to make life and death decisions all the time without help from anyone else. In fact, most junior jobs these days are well supported. A medical qualification is perhaps the most useful qualification you can have and the range of things that you can do with it is huge. Even the more familiar jobs of a surgeon, physician and psychiatrist are very different, as you will see later on in this book. Many people spend time in a hospital or GP practice before they apply to medicine to give them an idea of what a career in medicine is like. This can be extremely useful, particularly if you can observe a few doctors doing different jobs.

In recent years the career pathway for doctors has undergone a series of large changes. Gone are the days of House Officers and Registrars; these roles have been replaced with new and unfamiliar job titles like FY1 and StR. Many practising doctors get mixed up with these names so don't worry if they're new to you. Our comprehensive chapter on career paths explains why these changes came about and what all the new titles mean.

Understanding what a career in medicine is all about and how you will climb up the career ladder will help you to decide whether all the years of study are worth it. But what is medical school all about? Why is it so long? And how do you choose which one to go to? There are 31 medical schools in the UK and they all have their strengths and weaknesses. It is very hard to choose which ones to apply to, but a bit of knowledge about the different teaching styles and course structures will help you to narrow them down. For most, medical school is hugely enjoyable, both in terms of the course and social life. Seeing real patients (usually from the first year) gives a real taste for what being a doctor is all about. There is a variety to life as a medical student that you don't get in most other courses and an average week might include lectures, small group work, time on the wards talking to patients, and practise at clinical skills like how to take blood. Medical students form strong and lasting friendships as they share these exciting and unique experiences together.

One unwelcome consideration that puts many people off studying medicine is money. Five or more years without a regular or significant income can mean having to live a very humble existence – the average medical student loan exceeds

£20,000 at graduation. However, there are a variety of grants available for those unable to afford to go to medical school without assistance and with careful planning and some smart budgeting it should still be possible, as Chapter 7 explains.

Medicine is a unique career that opens up a huge range of opportunities. Few if any other careers can offer such a broad range of day-to-day activities and career paths. Being a doctor can be stressful, tiring, challenging, and sometimes upsetting but very rarely is it described as boring. It can be a real roller-coaster ride but is hugely rewarding. Deciding to embark on a career in medicine is a huge commitment though and is a big decision to make. I hope this book will help you to make the right one.

Good Luck!

Chapter 2 How do you ensure medicine is the right career for you?

Gayathri Rabindra

Medicine is a career that combines the intellectual demands and challenges of science with the satisfaction of helping others. It requires dedication and motivation, both at medical school and beyond. The shortest medical degree is four years long, and despite shorter working hours than in the past, working as a practising doctor is hard, involving long and antisocial hours. A medical career is therefore not something to be entered into lightly. Spending time researching what being a doctor involves is vital, not only to ensure that you are making an informed decision, but also to enhance your prospects of getting into medical school.

What do you want from your career?

Before we talk about medicine, let's talk about you. It is important to ask yourself some questions and speak to your friends, family and teachers. See if you can answer the following questions:

- What do you want from your career?
- What has made you think about becoming a doctor?
- What do you want to be doing in five, ten, or even 50 year's time?

Throughout this book you will read about the diversity of medicine as a career, how it can satisfy a wide range of personalities and interests. Having an idea of what you want from your career as you read on will help you to make up your mind.

What are you good at? What do you find a struggle?

People often enjoy jobs more when they are good at what they do. A medical degree opens up a wide variety of careers within medicine that appeal to different types of people. Medical school, junior doctor training and most specialties involve a lot of contact with people: patients, families, other doctors, nurses, pharmacists, physiotherapists, and so on. You don't have to be someone who loves every person who you've ever met to be a good doctor, but if you really don't like other people you might not enjoy it much.

Choosing a degree to study at university is incredibly daunting. It can be tempting to choose medicine as an 'easy option', so you can make the decision of degree and career in one and not have to decide anything else for many years.

If you enjoy science subjects at school and are considering medicine as an alternative to a career in scientific research, you should find out more about the life of a medical researcher. There are opportunities for combining medical training with academic research both at medical school and as a junior doctor. Contact a practising doctor who is involved in medical research and ask them about their job. Medical research is a huge field, with lots of opportunities to do research without a medical degree. Alternative degrees that could lead to medically related research include human sciences, life sciences, anatomy, physiology, neuroscience, and psychology.

Do you like routine or a lot of variety to your day?

There's not a lot of routine to the average working day of a doctor. If you don't like spontaneity then you might find being a doctor quite stressful.

What are the most important things to you in a career?

Is earning lots of money important to you? Try to be honest with yourself, as it is better to admit this sooner rather than later. In the later stages of your career your salary is good but this only comes after several years of training and antisocial hours – if money is your main priority then perhaps another career would be better for you.

Is job satisfaction important to you? For those who are suited to it, medicine offers this in abundance, and makes the long hours worth it.

Are you considering choosing medicine to please your parents or follow in their footsteps? This is a common reason why people choose medicine (even if they don't admit it). Although it is lovely to follow your parents' dreams, do make sure that you consider your own dreams and aspirations. A career in medicine is a huge commitment, and can be physically and emotionally draining. If you haven't chosen it for the right reasons, it will be even harder and you might find yourself more likely to drop out and not finish the course.

Do you have the qualities required to make a good doctor?

Do you want to help people? Do you have good communication skills? Are you able to work in a team? Can you make decisions under pressure? Different careers within medicine may require these qualities to greater or lesser degrees. Don't expect to be able to answer these questions all on your own – most people tend to be very critical of themselves when they think of things like this. So ask those close to you what they think.

So you think you're got what it takes to be a doctor – what next?

Next, you should find out more about what being a medical student and a doctor is really like. Talk to people you know who are doctors; your GP, relatives, friends, friends of friends or relatives of friends. Ask them to give you their viewpoint on life as a doctor. The more the better – so you can get as rounded a picture as possible. There is no substitute for work experience, as this will show you precisely what is involved in the day-to-day life of a doctor. If any other careers appeal to you, try to arrange to get some experience of those too.

It's also worth thinking early on about what you would need to do to apply for medical school.

When medical schools consider applications, they often have various academic and non-academic criteria in mind. Therefore it is important to find out well in advance what these criteria are (see Chapter 3). This can be done by looking at the individual prospectuses, and by attending open days at the universities that you are considering. Open days are an invaluable opportunity to meet current medical students and ask them questions. You also get a feel for the university and can try to imagine whether you would be happy to live there for the next few years.

Most people applying to medical school will have the required grades and academic credentials to achieve a place. Therefore it's really important not to underestimate how important the non-academic aspects of your application are. Extra-curricular activities help develop skills that will be useful in any career, but especially medicine. All UK medical schools tend to have similar non-academic requirements:

- Work Experience
- Teamwork
- Communication Skills
- Leadership/Responsibility
- Likely contribution to university life

As we look at some of these requirements in a little more detail, try not to think of them as hoops to jump through to get into medical school. Think about why they are so important to medical schools, and how being a doctor requires all of them to some degree.

Work experience

All medical schools want you to have some relevant work experience, and rightly so. It's only sensible to expect that students have some idea of the career that they are committing themselves to, and is invaluable in helping you decide whether medicine is really the career for you. You will gain experience of looking after patients and seeing first-hand whether this is something you enjoy. It is also an opportunity to look at the different career paths available within medicine, such as radiology and pathology, as well as more ward-based specialties. Remember, time spent researching a medical career now can save years of training if it turns out to be a career which you don't enjoy.

Your work experience doesn't have to be in a hospital – it can be difficult to find these opportunities. Any experience in a healthcare setting or 'helping people' is just as useful. Don't worry if a lot of what you see goes over your head; the purpose of work experience is not to learn the subject – after all, that's what medical school is for. It's more important for you to see what skills are involved in being a doctor. Look at how they deal with patients and colleagues, and what their daily work involves. Make sure you keep a note of your experiences and your reflections, as these can be useful to talk about at your interview. Try and put yourself in the doctor's shoes: can you see yourself doing their job in a few years time?

Most people think that practising medicine is hospital-based. However, a lot of it takes place in the community (known as 'primary care'), where general practitioners (GPs) play a key role.

Try and organise the work experience yourself. If you can say that you took the initiative this is much more impressive than if you tagged along with a relative for a day. Start early – there can be a lot of forms to fill in and people to contact before you can start your work experience, so avoid leaving it until the last minute. If you're finding it hard to find somewhere, here are some suggestions:

- Contact your local hospital. Most are accustomed to having work experience students and can advise you on the steps you need to take.

- Ask your general practitioner. It might not be possible to undertake work experience at your local practice, due to confidentiality issues, but they might put you in touch with one of their colleagues.

- Visit your school's careers advisor. They often have a database of doctors who have been willing to help in the past.

- Ask your relatives and friends if they know any doctors. It's better not to do work experience with them, but they may refer you to someone who can help.

- Try your local Connexions office (see www.connexions-direct.com)

Don't be disheartened if some people say no. People are generally willing to help even if they can't offer you a placement they might be able to suggest someone who can.

Voluntary work is often easier to become involved with and can be more useful than work experience. It shows your commitment and organisation, and demonstrates your caring side. Your options are endless, from volunteering in a hospital, hospice or nursing home, to working with disabled children in the community. Volunteering can be extremely rewarding, and is a great way for you to see what it's like working within the healthcare system. A commitment over a period of time looks better than a short burst, which can be interpreted by medical schools as being done just to add to your personal statement. You could even become a Millennium Volunteer and be recognised for the work you put in (see www.vinspired.com). Whatever you decide to do, make sure you reflect on your experiences and note down your thoughts. You can draw on these reflections when it comes to applying to medical school.

'I chose to work in play schemes with children with special needs, as I thought it would be relevant to medicine. I gained so much from it personally as well as professionally, and it really showed me that I wanted to be in a caring profession. In my interview the panel were really interested in my experiences and it was easy to talk about as I loved it.'

Teamwork

Medicine is full of teamwork. From dissecting a cadaver with your fellow students to working as a consultant with your colleagues trying to diagnose a complex case, you will be required to work in teams. For this reason, team-working skills are an essential requirement for entrance to medical school. There are many ways to show that you are a team player, such as playing in a sports team, being on a committee or organising an event.

Leadership skills

There may be opportunities for you to run societies or clubs at your school. Part-time jobs can also demonstrate commitment and responsibility. If you can't find a club that you're interested in, why not start one? Becoming a prefect or getting involved with mentoring schemes also give you the chance to improve your leadership skills.

The important thing is quality and not quantity: you don't have to list dozens of achievements or necessarily have reached a high standard. Nobody expects you to be the perfect leader or be able to make the correct decisions all the time. It is important, though, that you are willing to lead and make decisions and learn from these experiences.

Many people can talk about these skills from the hobbies and interests that they already have, so don't think you have to join hundreds of clubs and societies!

Extra-curricular activities

Medical schools are looking for well-rounded, sociable people who will contribute positively to medical school life. Extra-curricular activities demonstrate these things and show that you have good team-working, leadership and communication skills. During your working life you'll be doing long shifts and antisocial hours, so it's important that you have a good work/life balance.

Summary

Deciding that you want to become a doctor is one of the biggest decisions you are likely to make. It is vital that you enter into a career in medicine knowing what the job entails and that you have the motivation and skills to do it well. Try to get a taste for as many different aspects of medicine as possible before you apply. Then think about the qualities of a good doctor and whether you can prove that you have them. Look for any gaps in your experience and try to fill them before you apply.

Key points:

- Do plenty of research before deciding on a career in medicine

- Work experience is essential to your research: organise this early

- Once you've decided that you want to be a doctor, think about what medical school selectors are looking for

- Medical schools look at non-academic qualities to differentiate between applicants

- Demonstrate that you have good teamwork, leadership and communication skills

- Reflecting on your experiences is a great way to impress selectors.

Chapter 3 What steps are involved in the application process?

Gayathri Rabindra

Once you've decided that medicine is the career for you, you should turn your attention to the application process. In the UK this involves an entrance exam, UCAS (Universities and Colleges Admissions Service) application form and interview. The ratio of applicants to places is high and competition is fierce so you must stand out from the crowd, both academically and non-academically.

What are medical schools looking for?

The Council of Heads of Medical Schools issues guidance on the selection of students to medical schools. There are nine key principals.

- Selection for medical school implies selection for the medical profession.
- The selection process attempts to identify the academic and non-academic qualities of a doctor.
- A high level of academic attainment will be expected.
- The practice of medicine requires the highest standards of professional and personal conduct.
- The practice of medicine requires the highest standards of professional competence.
- Candidates should demonstrate some understanding of what a career in medicine involves and their suitability for a caring profession.

- Medical schools have agreed that the selection process must be transparent, and adhere to diversity and equality legislation.
- The primary duty of care is to patients.
- Failure to declare information that has a material influence on a student's fitness to practise may lead to termination of their medical course.

What does all of this mean for you? Well, in essence, when you apply for medical school you are also applying to become a doctor, which makes it unusual when compared to other degrees. Medical schools must be confident that every student they offer a place at medical school to is the right type of person to be a doctor. The previous chapter described many of the qualities of a doctor, but essentially they are looking for people who are well-rounded and caring, as well as academically strong. The application process aims to identify these people, so bear this is mind when preparing your interview and writing your personal statement.

Entrance exams

Increasing numbers of A-level students achieving top grades has made it difficult for admissions tutors to choose between the many thousands of applicants to medical school. This led to the development of entrance exams.

UKCAT (UK Clinical Aptitude Test) is the entrance exam required by most of the UK universities (www.ukcat.ac.uk). It is a test of aptitude rather than academic knowledge. The exam assesses five skills: verbal reasoning, quantitative reasoning, abstract reasoning, decision analysis and non-cognitive analysis. The exam is two hours long and can be taken at various dates between July and October, at different centres throughout the UK. Registration for the exam opens in May, and it is cheaper the earlier you book. Bursaries are available for certain students. Practice questions are available on the UKCAT website to give an idea of what to expect.

A few medical schools, namely Oxford, Cambridge, Imperial College and University College London, require the BMAT (BioMedical Admissions Test, www.bmat.org.uk). This exam consists of three papers testing aptitude and skills, scientific knowledge and applications, and a writing task. There is a mixture of multiple choice questions, short answer questions and short essays. It is only possible to sit the exam on one date each year so ensure you check about deadlines well in advance. In 2008 the exam was in November.

One student gives advice about preparation for the BMAT exam:

> *'I went over my GCSE science revision guides which were really useful since the questions aren't that taxing, they just require thinking outside the box. Past questions were the only way of preparing for the logic paper, to give an idea of what to expect. For the essay part I kept up-to-date with the news during the weeks running up to the BMAT and read up on the recent medical breakthroughs.'*

Revision books and further practice questions for the UKCAT and BMAT are also available at www.developmedica.com

The GAMSAT (Graduate Medical School Admissions Test) is the exam for certain graduate-entry programmes (www.gamsatuk.org). Like the BMAT, it is only offered once a year. It doesn't necessarily require a science background but does require some knowledge of biological and physical sciences. It tests concepts of basic science, as well as generic skills of problem-solving, critical thinking and writing.

It is essential that you research these exams early, as certain medical schools require different exams and have their own deadlines, some before the deadline for UCAS applications. You have to pay to take all the exams. In 2008 the UKCAT and BMAT exams cost £60 and £31 respectively. The fee to sit the GAMSAT is £195. All cost more if you register late.

The UCAS form

All medical school applications are made through UCAS. The UCAS form contains details about yourself and information from your teachers such as predicted grades and references. For most medical schools you will need predicted A-level grades of ABB or better. You can apply for up to six courses on your UCAS form, but you can only apply to four medical schools. You can leave the other two choices blank or apply for non-medical degrees.

The main part of the UCAS form which you have control over, and which determines whether you get shortlisted (as well as your grades and reference), is the personal statement.

The personal statement

This is your opportunity to show that you have what it takes to be a doctor and to really stand out from the crowd. You can be shortlisted or rejected outright at this stage, so make sure you sell yourself, catch their eye, and don't waste words.

Here are some tips for writing your personal statement.

- Have an engaging introduction and conclusion. These parts can make a good first impression and make sure you are remembered afterwards.
- Be concise.

- Use examples and reflect on what you learnt from your experiences.
- Allow your personality to shine through.
- Get opinions from other people. They don't need to have a medical background, as it can be useful to get their opinion about readability as well as content. Don't be upset or put off if you receive constructive criticism: the harsher people are now, the kinder your assessors will be further down the line!
- Tailor your personal statement to a career in medicine, even if you are also applying to non-medical courses.
- Don't make spelling and grammar mistakes.
- Don't go over the word limit or outside the box.
- Don't lie.
- Don't leave it until the last minute!

To start with, having that blank form in front of you is incredibly daunting. It can seem like you'll never be able to think of anything to write. But actually, the hardest part is deciding what not to write. It is easy to waffle but much harder to be crisp and concise. One way to improve your personal statement is to cut out anything that doesn't show that you fulfill the criteria for entry to medical school (make your own list of criteria using Chapter 2 and the prospectuses of the universities you are applying for). Once you've done that, look at what you've written and think how you could make it sound more impressive and concise.

Example from a personal statement:

> 'I want to study medicine as I like working with people. I spent a week at University College Hospital, a large teaching hospital, learning about cutting-edge techniques, such as laparoscopic

fundoplication. I volunteer with disabled children every week. I represent my school at tennis and swimming and compete in various tournaments. I run the Science Society at school and have been nominated to be a school prefect this year. I believe these experiences have given me the skills required to make a good doctor.'

This person obviously has a lot of achievements but it is difficult to get a sense that he understands what being a doctor involves. The listing-style is rather laborious to read and very little personality comes across. His comments about spending time at a world-leading hospital manage to sell the hospital rather than himself. The point of work experience is not to learn clever medicine, but to show you what the world of medicine is really about, so it's important that you state what you have learned from your experiences.

An improved version of the above would be:

'My work experience in a teaching hospital taught me about the significance of communication between doctor and patient to reach a diagnosis. I learnt the importance of a multi-disciplinary team in patient care. Volunteer work with disabled children has given me an intense sense of responsibility for those in need. Running the Science Society at school has improved my leadership skills and given me insight into effective team-working, which I think is incredibly important in medicine.'

In this version, you get a stronger a sense of what the student has learnt from their experience; they have made an effort to understand what it takes to be a doctor, rather than just passively observing. Reflection is really important in medicine – it helps you to learn from mistakes and is something that interview panels look for in a doctor.

As you fine-tune your personal statement, remember that it forms the basis for any interviews that you attend. Therefore, make sure that you are happy to discuss anything that you include on it – this will prevent difficulties later. For more help and advice regarding your personal statement visit www.developmedica.com

The interview

Most medical schools will interview prospective students prior to making offers. If you get to this stage then you have done extremely well – it shows that the tutors were impressed with your application so far and want to see more of you. So, once you receive an invitation to be interviewed, congratulate yourself, and then begin your preparation.

What does the interview involve? You should be told the format of the interview when you receive your invitation: some medical schools have just one interview, whilst others have two or three. If there is more than one interview then the subject matter may be different for each one; for example one may be more scientific and the other more general.

Expect your interview to last between 10 and 40 minutes. Most medical schools interview with a panel of tutors, medical students and lay people. There will probably be between two and four people on the panel. It is worth discussing with people who have had their interviews already or in previous years, but do remember that the questions are unlikely to be the same – the interviewers can and will ask you anything they like.

Practise, practise, practise! This may be the first interview you have had in your life, so it can be a very alien experience. The more you can practise, with friends, family and teachers, the less nerve-wracking the experience will be. Practise can also help identify things that you do without realising, such as nervous twitches or not making enough eye contact. Although it's useful to think of answers to common questions, don't learn answers by rote as it won't look genuine. Interview workshops can be useful, especially one that offers mock-interview practice.

On the day, make sure you dress professionally. You are going for an interview for entry into the medical profession, so make sure you look the part. Make sure though, that as well as looking smart, you feel comfortable in your interview clothes.

Now, down to the questions! They really can ask anything, but make sure you have thought about how you might answer the common ones. It's vital that you know your personal statement well, because you will be asked about it. Nothing looks worse than a student who gets stumped when asked about their work experience which they themselves chose to mention on their form!

'One of my interviews was purely based around my personal statement, with typical questions like "why medicine?" and "what have you gained from voluntary work and work experience?" They also gave me a scenario which said I had to break bad news to a patient who had cancer and I had to describe how I would go about it.'

Make sure you learn about the medical school where you are being interviewed, including the course structure and any extra-curricular activities on offer that interest you. This demonstrates you have really researched the course, and shows the panel that you have something to offer them.

'Why do you want to be a doctor?'

This is the most obvious question to ask, so do think about it beforehand. Hopefully, you will have thought about this whilst brainstorming for your personal statement. Don't get yourself worked up about it, as it is a difficult question to answer without sounding cheesy or repetitive; the chances are that the panel have heard it all before. Use the opportunity to show that you know what skills are required and that you have thought about whether you fit the criteria. You could expand your answer by backing it up with examples, such as from your work experience.

Many questions will be 'open questions', such as 'tell us about your work experience?' This might make you relax as you know you can talk about whatever you like, but this is the worst attitude to have. Remember, the interviewers want you to show them that you have the right qualities to be a doctor – make sure you sell yourself and show that you have reflected on your experiences.

Topical questions are another common question so make sure you prepare for these. The easiest way to do this is to read health news in newspapers or online. When asked about a topical issue at interview, show that you understand the pros and cons, and can form a reasonable opinion by yourself. So if you are asked 'what do you think of euthanasia?' – don't just wade in with 'it's bad'. Talk about what you understand about euthanasia, why some people are in favour of it and others against, then state your thoughts. Also try and have an idea about the NHS and career structures (see Chapter 10).

What if you don't know what to say? It is much better to say that you don't know than to waffle on for ages and dig yourself into a hole. Equally, if you keep saying 'I don't know about that topic' then it doesn't look good either, so it really is important to do some preparation!

Most interviews end with the interviewers asking if you have any questions for them. Don't panic about this, it's better not to ask a question than to ask something that could have been found out from the prospectus or at an open day. If you do have a question that you would like to ask, don't be afraid to, but saying something like 'all my questions have been answered by the prospectus and open day' will do fine. There is further help and advice on how to succeed in your interview available at www.developmedica.com

Summary

Medical schools have a responsibility to select suitable students for their courses. They have guidelines to help them indentify suitable candidates. When you are filling out your application form and preparing for interviews try to keep these guidelines in mind and relate all of your experience and interests to these. Prove to them that you are what they are looking for and you will succeed.

Key points:

- Find out about entrance exam and UCAS deadlines early

- Make your personal statement reflective and concise

- Practise is key to a successful interview

- Know your personal statement inside out for your interview.

Chapter 4 How to choose which medical school to apply for

Matthew Harrison

Choosing which medical school to apply to is one of the most difficult aspects of your application. Even though there are 31 medical schools to choose from, you may feel that they all seem to be offering roughly the same thing. A read through the prospectuses might not get you much closer to deciding which one is right for you. They each talk about their teaching style, intercalation, clinical training and boast about their extra-curricular activities, but they might not say a lot about the location of the medical school, how far you have to travel, or the cost of living locally. This chapter will discuss these aspects, to help you make a shortlist of your favourites and think of questions to ask when you visit them.

The course

There are three types of medical course: undergraduate courses for those who haven't yet been to university; graduate courses for those who already have a degree; and foundation (or access) courses for those who don't have the grades or are from a non-science background. An undergraduate course lasts for five years, or six if you decide to intercalate. Graduate-only courses are usually shorter and therefore can be more intense. Teaching styles may also be different. A couple of universities do not allow graduates onto the undergraduate course, so be sure to check with them before applying if this applies to you.

Teaching style

Broadly speaking, there are two types of medical course: traditional lecture-based and problem-based learning (PBL for short) courses. PBL is a relatively new style of teaching, and it tends to be used more by the newer medical schools. Traditional lecture-based teaching is popular with the more established medical schools though some of these also use PBL and many like to mix the two.

Traditional teaching, as the name implies, is the way it's always been done: students go to lectures and attend practical lessons (such as dissection). They progress in a stepwise manner learning the basic science of medicine, building an understanding of diseases and how to treat them upon this.

PBL teaches medicine in a different manner. As the name suggests, students are given 'problems' – usually information about a patient with a particular disease – and then they have to work their way backwards, with guidance of course, to the science underpinning that disease.

Both of these methods have their advantages and disadvantages and they both seem to produce equally capable doctors, so which one you choose comes down mainly to personal preference. Students who like to work independently and have no difficulty motivating themselves often prefer PBL – it is far more engaging than sitting in lectures listening to someone drone on about the anatomy of the kidney! You tend to work in small groups, which can be very enjoyable. Indeed, many people say that the group work that is involved in problem-based learning prepares you very well for being a doctor. On the other hand, the great thing about lectures is that you know that the lectures will cover most, if not all, of what will be in your exams.

It is worth bearing in mind that there is no clear line between traditional and problem-based learning – most medical schools with lecture-based courses have quite a bit of PBL in the course, and all PBL courses will have some lectures too.

Intercalation
Anyone who has an interest in academic medicine or research should certainly consider the possibility that they might want to do an intercalated BSc when choosing where to apply to. It can also help when applying for jobs and it looks good on a CV, especially if the degree is in a related topic to the job you are applying for (e.g. Neuroscience for aspiring Neurologists). For others, an intercalated year is just another year without an income or a 50,000 word dissertation that they could do without. See Chapter 8 for more about intercalation.

Location
A lot of what you feel when you look around a university for the first time depends on how likeable the area or city is. Do not be put off or influenced too much by this though. Speaking to current students at the open day will give you a good insight into what the area's like. In some places, particularly London, many students choose to live away from the main campus after their first year to save money – try to ask someone about this, how long it takes to get to lectures and how much travel will cost.

Town or country
There are no medical schools in the countryside but there are some in smaller cities or on the outskirts of cities rather than located in the centre. What you choose really comes down to personal preference. Some like a peaceful semi-rural location

while others like all the hustle and bustle of a busy city centre. During your last couple of years at medical school you are very likely to have to spend some time at smaller hospitals in the towns and suburbs around your medical school.

Joint schools

Some medical schools operate as a partnership between two universities and the year group is split between two sites. If this is the case, get a good feel for both universities as you could be based at either.

Proximity to home

For many people going to university will be their first time away from home. Living away is part of the university experience, and many advise that you should move out of home if you can. But you shouldn't dismiss a medical school just because it is close to your home – there's little sense in traveling halfway across the country to a university when there's a better one on your doorstep. For some people being close to home may be important and you may have family or other commitments that you simply cannot leave – don't worry if this applies to you, as you won't be the only day scholar on the course. The disadvantage of being at home is that you could feel more isolated from the rest of the university, but there's no reason why that has to be the case. Being in your own home does have its advantages, especially if there is someone there to cook dinner after a long afternoon in lectures.

Cost of living

Unfortunately, going to university costs money and this needs to be taken into account when choosing which medical school to apply to. Outgoings such as rent in any university city can be quite high, but some places are more expensive than others. The obvious example is London, where private rentals are usually over £100 per week (although halls of residences are usually cheaper and you will receive a bigger loan to help cover this). Chapter 7 has more information on living costs. Generally the further away from London the cheaper it is – and no, the Faroe Islands don't have a medical school!

Going Private

Whilst we're on the subject of living costs, this might be a good time to mention the option of studying abroad at a private medical school. There are several medical schools outside the UK that offer medical degree courses to British students. The main ones are Charles University in Prague and St Matthews University on the Cayman Islands. The cost of living in these places is significantly lower than the UK and living in the Caribbean does have other advantages. The main problem with private schools is the fees, which currently stand at between £8,000 and £11,000 per year for Charles University and about £9,000 per semester for St Matthews.

There are plans to open a private medical school in the UK. What its role will be in UK medical education is not yet clear and at the time of writing the General Medical Council will not register graduates from UK-based private medical schools.

Specific requirements

It is worth checking whether any of the medical schools that you are applying to have any specific requirements for applicants. You need to consider whether you need to sit the BMAT or UKCAT entrance exams (see Chapter 3). You should also check what A-levels are required and the typical grades that are needed for entry.

Competition

Just because places at a particular medical school are very competitive doesn't mean you shouldn't apply there. Having said that you shouldn't ignore competition completely, so you need to get the balance right between applying for the medical schools that you really want to go to, and being realistic about your chances of getting in. Studying competition ratios can be useful as they give you an idea of which medical schools are more popular with applicants. Looking at last year's ratios will not tell you what this year's will be like, but they will give you a rough idea. Some people don't apply to their first choice of medical school because they think it is too competitive. Consider this carefully because when it comes to the interview, your desire to go to that medical school will shine through and increase your chances of being accepted dramatically.

Reputation

There are various league tables that attempt to rank medical schools according to the quality of the course, job prospects, student life and so on. These league tables are taken very seriously by the medical schools as a low position can affect the quality of their applicants. Reputation is built on other things too, such as academic research and famous alumni. Medical schools with a better reputation don't necessarily produce better doctors, so don't put too much emphasis on it.

Some British universities have names that are recognised across the world. If you can say on your CV that you have a degree from Oxford or Cambridge you may well have an advantage when it comes to jobs. Universities with good academic or clinical reputations may also give better opportunities to their students – they are often connected to high quality research centres, so if you feel on your course that you want to delve deeper into a particular field you'll be in the perfect place to do it.

University or Medical School

These two terms are used interchangeably and so they should be – medical schools are part of universities! But it may surprise you to know that in some places the medical school is more of a part of the university than in others. Many medical schools have their own set of clubs and societies and you may find that in some cases these have little contact with those of the rest of the university. In some places the medical school may even operate almost as a completely separate enclave within the university where medical students have their own clubs, bars, societies, football leagues, choirs and everything else for that matter; contact with the rest of the university is minimal. In other places the medical school is as integrated into university life as any other department and medical students are just as much part of the university as anybody else. This is particularly the case in universities that maintain a college system, as ties to your college are as strong as to your school.

Wherever you go you might find that to some degree medics do tend to stick together. This is due to a number of factors. Firstly, the course length means that many of your friends on other courses in the first year will leave when you finish your third year, leaving you to do another year or two with the rest of the medics. Secondly, the location of the medical school may be away from the university's main campus. Medical schools are often attached to university hospitals. These can be geographically isolated from the rest of the university, making keeping in touch with what is happening difficult.

Another reason why it can be hard not to spend all your time with other medical students is the structure of the course. As well as having more hours of lectures and seminars than most other courses, exam dates for medical students are usually different to the rest of the university. With all of these barriers to making friends with so-called 'non-medics', it is easy to see why medical students have a reputation for being cliquey.

Summary

Every university has its own peculiarities and character and every medical school has its own allegiances and rivalries. There is a rich and varied selection to choose from. Like chocolate, no matter how many people you ask to help you choose, or how many times you read that little card that comes with them, you're never going to know what they're really like until you try them. Also like chocolate, the one that looks the best to you is the one that you're going to enjoy the most.

Key points:

- There are a variety of medical schools both in the UK and abroad

- Go on open days long before you apply and obtain as much information as you can

- Weigh up the pros and cons of your choices carefully and go for what feels best

- Wherever you go you're bound to have fun.

Chapter 5 What is life like as a medical student?

Matthew Harrison

Medicine isn't so much a course but a lifestyle. Studying medicine is very rewarding and you never stop learning. This chapter gives an overview of what you can expect, and some tips on what to do and how to prepare.

Once you have accepted an offer from a medical school you will inevitably receive guidelines on how and what to prepare for medical school.

Injections

You will need to make sure that all your booster injections are up-to-date and provide the dates of when you last had them to the occupational health department. You will also need to schedule your Hepatitis B vaccination, which is a course of three vaccinations and involves having your antibody levels checked. Your medical school will send you exact details of what you need to do. Once you receive their letter, arrange an informal discussion with your GP (who are always helpful and supportive of medical students).

Books

Your reading list is likely to be extensive, but do not purchase any of the books yet. Your course could be based on a particular textbook, and whilst some books will be essential others may be totally unnecessary. The 'second years' can tell you which books to buy and which not to buy and they may even have an old copy for you. If you want to make a start with your reading list, then you could buy a generic anatomy or physiology textbook, for example:

- Kumar, P. and Clark, M. (2005) *Kumar and Clark Clinical Medicine*, Saunders, London;
- Koeppen, B. and Stanton, B. (2008) *Berne and Levy Physiology*, Mosby, Philadelphia;
- Pocock, G. and Richards, C. (2006) *Human Physiology: the basis of medicine*, Oxford University Press, Oxford;
- Drake, R. Vogl, W. and Mitchell, A. (2004) *Gray's Anatomy for students*, Churchill Livingstone, London;
- Moore, K. and Dalley, A. (2005) *Clinically Orientated Anatomy*, Lippincott Williams and Wilkins, Baltimore;
- Tortora, G. (2005) *Principles of Anatomy and Physiology*, John Wiley and Sons, Denver.

These are some examples of general textbooks; the best advice is still to wait as you may happen to find one in a charity shop. The concepts behind Anatomy or Physiology change little so it doesn't really matter if you buy older editions.

Equipment
The only piece of kit you are likely to need is a stethoscope. A white coat used to be an essential item but policy has changed regarding these, so whether you need one or not will vary between hospitals. In both cases there are often offers on during freshers' week where you could find a bargain; there are also websites where medical students can purchase these items at a reduced price, so you are unlikely to save money by purchasing them beforehand.

Accommodation

Having suitable accommodation is essential (unless of course you're living at home). Whilst universities usually guarantee a room to all 'first years', there can, however, be a variation in quality. Halls accommodation is often allocated on a first come, first served basis, and as a medical student you may be lucky as you receive your offers earlier than. Some establishments may remove this advantage by preventing you from applying for accommodation until a later date when all students will have received their offers. In any case it is important to know what you want and to apply early. You don't need to accept what is on offer from the university, so keep your options open. It could be difficult finding a house to share in your first year as you probably won't know anyone but there are always rooms going if you look around. Another accommodation option is using a private hall of residence. These do tend to be more expensive but they are generally of a higher quality.

Other things to take

Check what you need in your accommodation: some provide everything, some nothing. You will easily be able to check this when you have your accommodation offer. Where clothing is concerned, remember to take something clinically suitable. For men, a shirt and trousers (tie policy varies), and for women it's a little more difficult; needless to say it must be smart and not too revealing. You won't have to wear this day-to-day, but if you need to see a patient you will have to be smart. The only other thing to consider here is transport. In the first year it probably isn't necessary to own a car but as you start placements later on in the course it becomes more and more useful to have one. This obviously depends on the geographical area your medical school covers and the provision of public transport.

Freshers' week

In your first year of medical school you are a 'fresher'. The first week of the year is known as 'freshers' week', and for many students this mainly consists of parties and plenty of alcohol. However, as a medical student things might be slightly different. You will probably have to enrol on your course on the Monday of freshers' week; don't be surprised if lectures start straight away. Most other courses start the week after freshers' week, or in some cases even the week after that. Your course starts as soon as you arrive. That doesn't mean to say that there won't be parties; there will be and you will soon discover that medical students know how to enjoy themselves!

If partying isn't your scene then don't worry, there are plenty of other things to do. Whilst your flatmates may not need to leave their rooms for several days, you are likely to need to attend lectures. There will be other, more mundane things to do in freshers' week: having your picture taken perhaps multiple times for all manner of ID cards; registering with the university's occupational health department; handing in your immunisation record and having blood taken; also you will need to register with a GP. These are all likely to be timetabled into your teaching.

One of the most important things to do during freshers' week is to go to the freshers' fayre. This is the place where all the societies and clubs of the university sell their wares. Some medical schools have their own fayre, but even so try to go to the main one as well, it's a good chance to see what the university is all about and meet other students from outside your course. There will be every club you can possibly imagine but resist the temptation to join them all. Most clubs will offer a trial period of membership which you can sample for the first couple of weeks and join up later. There will also be a plethora of freebies available so be sure to get what you can (free pens are especially useful).

There are a few essentials for freshers' week.

- Paperwork sent to you by the university; you'll need it to register.
- Cheque book (but don't be too frivolous with them).
- Note-taking materials; your lectures will start immediately.
- Well groomed face and hair: you picture will be on your ID badge for the next five years.

After freshers' week

Once the blur of freshers' week has passed and you feel you may just have recovered from all the excitement, you may or may not be looking forward to making a start. What you will actually be doing is covered in Chapter 8. The rest of this chapter is concerned with advice about other things.

Managing your time effectively

You've come through GCSEs, A-Levels and possibly another degree if you're a graduate, so you have some idea about what your time management skills are like. It's hard to suggest what to do with your time because different things work for different people, but here are some general tips:

- Try and find out where you need to be and when. A diary can be useful as although you are likely to be given a timetable, it might be a large format and practically impossible to understand.
- Try to be organised with your notes. This is much easier said than done – it is said that studying medicine is like trying to

drink water from a fire hose. It's good to try and keep on top of your notes otherwise they will quickly overwhelm you. File them or have somewhere to put them, even if it's just a box on your bedroom floor – at least you'll know where they are when it comes to revision.

- Start revision early: the earlier the better. You may not find the things you learn at medical school harder than at A-Level, but there will definitely be much more of it. You might have more notes from your first term that you did from your entire A-Level course, and a good revision plan will tell you how long it will take you to get through your notes. Another important thing to remember about medical exams is that you can't know everything. This may be distressing for some of you who are used to knowing everything that you need to know – you may have to be satisfied with just knowing enough.

Budgeting

This will be covered in detail in Chapter 7 so only a brief mention here. One good aspect of medicine is that there are very few course costs (compared to other subjects like art) where you have a lot of materials to buy. Your main expense for the course will be books. Textbooks usually cost between £20 and £50 each, generally speaking. The trick is to only buy what you absolutely need. If you're clever you can get through medical school with only two or three textbooks; carefully select the ones most appropriate to your course and the ones that suit you best. Some recommend buying books between groups. This does save on cost but can be more difficult when you all want the book leading up to an exam. Your only other costs will be extra-curricular and it's down to you to manage those wisely.

Facilities available to you

We can't of course tell you everything you can expect to have access to at every medical school, but there are some things that are common to most.

Faculty/Course Office

This should be your first port of call if you feel yourself needing help. The office staff will be able to give you a hand with a multitude of things and if they can't help you they're bound to know someone who can. Make sure you know where the course office is and if all else fails go there.

Library

Every medical school will have a library and you will no doubt be introduced to it in your first week. Medical libraries contain almost every book you could ever possibly want; unfortunately they never have enough copies of every book for every student. If you want to borrow one of the core textbooks you might have to move quickly. Many libraries now sign up to e-books; these are useful as you'll be able to access them wherever you are via the internet.

IT

As well as the library, medical schools often have separate, dedicated computer suites dotted around the place. You will have access to the university network, which has a selection of useful resources. There will also be internet access. It's handy to find these suites; sometimes they're well hidden but tend not to be as busy as the main libraries. As well as information available on the internet, universities also subscribe to additional materials that you can access. These might be e-books or e-journals, or perhaps specialist medical search engines or teaching packages.

Clinical Skills Labs

This is where you are likely to learn clinical skills such as how to take blood, insert a catheter and listen for heart murmurs. As well as timetabled sessions, the clinical skills lab usually has 'drop in' sessions where you can practise whatever you feel like.

Extra-curricular activities

You will be pleased to know that medical school isn't all study and that extra-curricula activities outside medicine form an important part of the degree. Not only will they help you to remain a well-rounded individual whilst studying, they are also a lot of fun.

The Medical Society and Students Union

Many of the events in freshers' week are organised by your students union or medical society. They also organise other activities throughout the year such as balls, charity fundraisers, open mic evenings and many other events. Membership of the Medical Society will get you cheap or free entry to most of their events as well as discounts on other things.

The Medical Society may also act as the co-ordinator for other medical societies; these cover a wide range of things from rugby, tennis and football to religious and debating societies, all within the medical school.

The students union are the people to turn to if you've anything political to get off your chest, and are always running campaigns in the interests of the student body. Medics will have representatives on the union and these are the people to contact. They organise feedback and complaints that can be taken to the medical school board. They also have pastoral support schemes and can give advice about almost any aspect of student life. The students union is a great thing to get involved in and can nurture any political aspirations you may have.

Sports

Think of a sport, any sport, and whatever it is the chances are you'll be able to do it at university. The more common sports such as swimming, football, rugby, tennis and cricket are always played (or swum). There is also likely to be every other sport you could possibly imagine: diving, fencing, pot-holing, paragliding and even tiddlywinks.

University is a great place to take up a new sport and the way to find the clubs is through the freshers' fayre. All the clubs will be keen to have you even if you've never had a go before. Once you're signed up all you've got to do is find the time and money to do it. Obviously this varies between sports; a diving kit or a paraglider will cost more than football boots or a set of dominoes!

Societies

There are numerous societies to join, too numerous to list, but they cover everything from religion and politics, fan clubs, food and travel, drama, or stamp collecting to historical re-enactment. Whatever your interests there'll be something for you. You may find yourself enjoying something you never thought you would and before you know it you'll be on a bus trip to the 'Stockport Museum of Hatting' having joined the Headwear Appreciation Society.

Support

We all need support to prevent things going wrong and to sort them out if they do. Medical schools realise that studying can be stressful at times and therefore do everything they can to support you.

Medic families

These are run by a number of medical schools as a way of ensuring that you will get support from the students in the years above you. Soon after arriving, you will be introduced to a second year student, your 'medic parent'. They should be able to tell you all you need to know about the year ahead, what to do, and what books to buy – they might even have an old textbook for you. In turn, they will also have a parent in the third year; your 'medic grandparent' who will be able to tell you even more. Somewhere in fifth year, (if you seek them out), will be your 'medic great, great grandparent'. Like any family some medic families are closer than others and some are even dysfunctional – there may be an adoption service for children or parents feeling they need more.

Tutors

Your tutor will be a member of clinical or academic staff who will act as your official pastoral support. During your first couple of years you will have fairly regular contact with your tutor. They should be your first point of contact if you need help or to discuss anything personal. They'll talk through your exam results with you and will be able to help you to get in touch with the university's counselling service or have extenuating circumstances taken into account when exams are being marked.

Summary

We can't pretend that you'll enjoy every aspect of your medical course for the whole five years. But for every little bit that irritates you there'll be something else you adore. Whatever your life as a medical student is like, it will affect your entire future and your time at university will probably be the most enjoyable you ever have.

Key points:

- Be sure to find out what you need to arrange before starting medical school, and ensure your vaccinations are up to date.

- Don't buy any books before you start.

- Your lectures are likely to begin in freshers' week so don't expect a gentle start.

- Be involved with activities outside the course; they will keep you sane even in the midst of exams.

- If you do need help, ask for it.

Chapter 6 Mature or graduate entry medicine – what is it all about?

Catherine Cheesman

We are currently in a period of unprecedented access to medical schools in terms of age, background and eligibility. Equally, competition for places has risen apace. Since 1997, places at medical school have risen from 5,000 to 7,500 per year. The increase in access is partly a reflection of wider changes in society, and latterly with a government initiative to widen access to medicals schools. Many of the new places at medical schools are going to so called 'mature students' who are beyond school leaving age. Mature students have found favour with medical schools as they are seen to be more single-minded, are less likely to drop out (or be thrown out), have valuable life-skills, and may be quicker and cheaper to train.

There is no doubt that studying medicine at any age should not be embarked on with flippancy. For the mature entrant facing the Himalayan peaks of preparation for eligibility, the application process and years of short-sight inducing study requires a dogged certainty that you are pursuing the right career. This chapter aims to help you determine whether you have what it takes by encouraging you to think about what graduate medical courses are really about and what the application process involves. It should act as a springboard for you to discover in more detail about each graduate entry medical course, so if you decide to apply for one you will have the greatest chances of success.

So, what is it all about?

Graduate entry is distinct from studying medicine as a mature student on an undergraduate course, although all may finish up on the same course for the clinical years. Graduate entry programmes (GEPs) and standard undergraduate courses will both lead to you becoming a doctor and securing provisional registration with the GMC – although the letters after your name may be different depending on which medical school you go to (see UCAS or individual prospectus listings).

Graduate entry programmes

Most of these dedicated courses are accelerated and take four years in total. Typically, the pre-clinical part of the course is separate from that of the undergraduate course of five years. For the clinical years, graduate entry courses and undergraduate courses are often the same.

Graduate entry courses are intense, with shorter holidays and require a high degree of motivation and self-directed learning. They frequently use problem-based learning (PBL) and inter-active styles, and are usually integrated to give early clinical experience. Both science and non-science graduates may be accepted, but this varies according to the institution. Usually a BSc (Hons) science degree is required. Most expect a minimum of a 2:1, although some schools accept a 2:2, particularly if you have a post-graduate qualification (PhD or MSc). The Open University has a specific course to upgrade a 2:2 degree to a 2:1 (see the Open University website at the end of the chapter). A health related degree or extenuating circumstances for your 2:2 may be accepted by some medical schools. Be aware that some medical schools stating a 2:1 as minimum are so over-subscribed that they may only select those with 1st class degrees. In practice, an average cohort is a third with 1sts and two thirds with 2:1s. Some GEPs specify A-level requirements too, but the main factor that determines whether or not you get an interview is your score on the GAMSAT or other entrance exam.

'The intensity of the course is a whole order higher than in, for example, a humanities degree so your previous academic experience may be just a warm-up really.'

GAMSAT

GAMSAT is short for the Graduate Australian Medical School Admissions Test. It is required at medical schools such as St. George's, Nottingham/Derby, Swansea and Peninsula (five year course). It comprises an arduous set of three exams over five hours. Each exam tests a different attribute that you need to have to become a good doctor:

- Reasoning – social sciences and humanities (75 MCQs).
- Communicative ability (two essays).
- Scientific reasoning. The exam is 40 per cent chemistry, 40 per cent biology and 20 per cent physics at or above an A-level standard (110 MCQ).

The GAMSAT website has more details on each of these exams. It is usually sat in September and in 2008 cost £195. The result is valid for entry within two years. You will need to revise for these exams – past papers are available, as are coaching courses but these can be costly.

'I diffidently sent off for some past papers and bought some basic science primers, which I assiduously studied for around four months before taking the exam. In fact, I enjoyed the studying for its own sake, it had been so long since I'd really applied myself to anything so purely academic. To be honest, I

never seriously thought that I'd do well enough in the exam to get an interview and I definitely didn't feel that I'd done particularly well on the day. Roughly, when you sit the GAMSAT you will probably be in a huge hall with several hundred other hopefuls (and don't forget the two thousand or so others in various other venues) who your nerves tell you are no doubt much more intelligent than you are. I was stunned, literally, when the results came in and I was in the 90th percentile. Before that I hadn't really believed that I was scientifically clever enough to be a doctor. Unfortunately, by that point it was too late to do any practical preparation for the interview e.g. do some work in the healthcare sector. Therefore I was turned down at interview.

For various reasons I let a year slide by before re-applying. The second time I took an AS level in human biology, worked for a few months as a carer, took a first aid course and volunteered at a clinical trial. So the second time around I was pretty serious about getting into medical school and I knew what I needed to do to that end. Taking the GAMSAT was more or less the same in results but a lot easier to do in terms of preparation and the sitting of the thing itself, basically because I wasn't intimidated anymore.'

Several GEPs require either the BMAT or UKCAT exams. For more information about these see Chapter 3.

Mature entry medicine

GEPs are not the only way for mature students to get into medical school. You can also apply to the standard five (or six) year undergraduate programmes. Many medical schools have a small quota of places reserved for mature students, although some do not allow graduates onto their undergraduate course, preferring them to apply to their GEPs (Nottingham and

St. George's are examples). Without a degree, application to undergraduate courses requires good science A-level grades. The minimum GCSE requirements are also the same. If you have non-science A-levels, lower grades, or if you have not studied in the last three years, you might consider taking more A-levels or an access course. A-levels can be taken part-time over a year at a local further education college. Access courses are not generally seen as another route past re-sits (which some medical schools are put off by). They are usually full-time for a year, and have fees (there are loans and bursaries available to help you pay for these). Access courses are generally for those that do not have science A-levels, have previously pursued other careers, or have come from a background that may have prejudiced their chances of entry into medicine. They are not a medical qualification, and although an increasing number of medical schools recognise them, not all of them do. Some offer a small number of guaranteed places onto their medical degree course (Leeds offer five places for example), but generally they do not. High marks are usually needed if you are to get into medical school afterwards, and you will have to sit the same entrance examinations as other applicants.

Six year foundation courses also provide another potential escape route from having to study science A-levels for those who have good non-science A-levels and want to get into medicine.

How do I decide which course to apply to?

Any uncertainty about your suitability or lack of work experience must be resolved before you apply to medical school (see Chapter 3). Discuss your application with people you trust will give you objective views, as you will need concise and eloquent promotion of your uniqueness both in your personal statement and at interview. Talk to others about your past employment, experiences and volunteer work and think about how they will help you in your medical career. You need strong selling points, especially if you are older.

Age

Many schools do not have an upper age limit, and there are plenty of 'forty-somethings' and a sprinkling of over fifties currently studying medicine. Careers options, pre-retirement employment time and general fitness may be factors you need to weigh up personally. You need to be able to endure the late nights of study, followed by the long shifts, weekends and on-call work.

Partner/family

Returning to full-time study, particularly if you are a wage-earner, has long term implications for a partner or family. It may be that you have to relocate, down-size, move to rented accommodation, or take out loans; your partner may also have to change jobs or hours. All of this can cause tension, especially if you have not made a considered and long-term plan. Mortgage, childcare costs, and holidays that don't coincide with school holidays must also be considered. Some medical schools allow parents to adjust a rotation so that holiday time overlaps that of family, but no extra time can be taken off due to the relentless nature of the curriculum. Being prepared is important because you cannot expect preferential treatment because of your circumstances. That said, crises can occur and most medical schools have very good systems in place for students with health problems, family issues or any other concerns (e.g. sporting commitments).

Geographical location/ relocation

You may choose to apply to medical schools nearby, but if you have to apply further afield, your choices are limited to where you are prepared to move. If you have a family, schooling choices may be a factor. Relocation means uprooting from family, social and recreational spheres, and may require greater effort to stay connected.

Finance

Tuition fees currently stand at £3,070 per year. You can obtain maintenance loans to help you cover some of these costs, and as a graduate entrant you can get an NHS Bursary for your second, third and fourth years. You may be allowed to spread the cost of tuition fees for the first year. Note that if UK graduates apply for an undergraduate course, as from September 2006, they cannot obtain a student loan for the tuition fees of a second degree, so will have to pay these upfront.

If you are very prudent and hardworking, you may be able to save up a lump sum that will keep you out of debt throughout medical school. More commonly though, people live on a shoestring, take out loans, work a few hours, take placements offering free accommodation in outlying hospitals, and pay off the debt later.

'I had a five-year plan to get in to medicine, I saved money and I worked as an auxiliary nurse for two years.'

Studying with school leavers

This is largely down to character and sociability, but you may find that if you are older, it can be hard to make a connection with some undergraduate students. Keep an open mind and try to remember how you felt when you were an 18 years old!

Mature

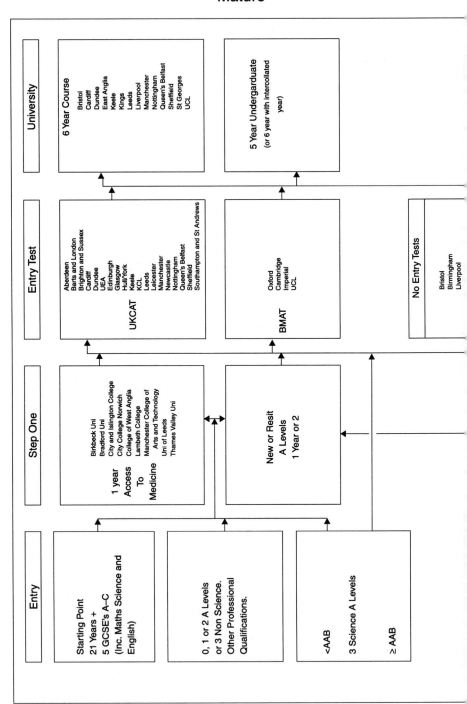

Entry	Step One	Entry Test	University

Entry

Starting Point
21 Years +
5 GCSE's A–C
(Inc. Maths Science and English)

0, 1 or 2 A Levels
or 3 Non Science.
Other Professional Qualifications.

<AAB

3 Science A Levels

≥ AAB

Step One

1 year Access To Medicine

Birkbeck Uni
Bradford Uni
City and Islington College
City College Norwich
College of West Anglia
Lambeth College
Manchester College of Arts and Technology
Uni of Leeds
Thames Valley Uni

New or Resit
A Levels
1 Year or 2

Entry Test

UKCAT

Aberdeen
Barts and London
Brighton and Sussex
Cardiff
Dundee
UEA
Edinburgh
Glasgow
Hull/York
Keele
KCL
Leeds
Leicester
Manchester
Newcastle
Nottingham
Queen's Belfast
Sheffield
Southampton and St Andrews

BMAT

Oxford
Cambridge
Imperial
UCL

No Entry Tests

Bristol
Birmingham
Liverpool

University

6 Year Course

Bristol
Cardiff
Dundee
East Anglia
Keele
Kings
Leeds
Liverpool
Manchester
Nottingham
Queen's Belfast
Sheffield
St Georges
UCL

5 Year Undergarduate
(or 6 year with intercollated year)

Graduate

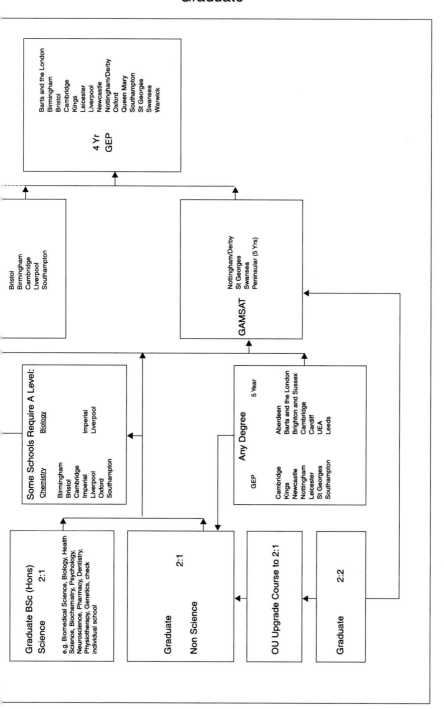

Graduate BSc (Hons)
Science   2:1

e.g. Biomedical Science, Biology, Health Science, Biochemistry, Psychology, Neuroscience, Pharmacy, Dentistry, Physiotherapy, Genetics, check individual school

Some Schools Require A Level:

Chemistry   Biology

Birmingham   Imperial
Bristol   Liverpool
Cambridge
Imperial
Liverpool
Oxford
Southampton

Bristol
Birmingham
Cambridge
Liverpool
Southampton

4 Yr
GEP

Barts and the London
Birmingham
Bristol
Cambridge
Kings
Leicester
Liverpool
Newcastle
Nottingham/Derby
Oxford
Queen Mary
Southampton
St Georges
Swansea
Warwick

Graduate
Non Science   2:1

Any Degree   5 Year

GEP

Cambridge   Aberdeen
Kings   Barts and the London
Newcastle   Brighton and Sussex
Nottingham   Cambridge
Leicester   Cardiff
St Georges   UEA
Southampton   Leeds

GAMSAT

Nottingham/Derby
St Georges
Swansea
Peninsular (5 Yrs)

OU Upgrade Course to 2:1

Graduate
2:2

You might have the opportunity to test how you deal with this unusual problem by taking an A-level at a local college, or when you attend university open days. This is rarely a major problem though, since there are always plenty of other mature students to hang around with and there are lots of opportunities, on firms and in seminars, to get to know other students on a more personal level.

Timing

You may be desperate to get on with your application as fast as you can, knowing that there are many long years of study ahead. For some though, it may be prudent to take time out to do other qualifications, study, or obtain experience to give yourself the best marketable chance of acceptance into medical school. Some medical schools limit you to two or three attempts, but others can refuse you further attempts after a single application on suitability grounds. If you have a long-term partner, and want a family some day, this needs to be factored in to your decision.

Application

Using all four UCAS choices for GEP courses has been considered risky due to the competition. Numbers of applicants per place do vary considerably, with over 60 applicants per place at one London university one year, compared to five per place elsewhere. Competition ratios are very variable, and you can check the statistics on-line (e.g. www the medschoolsonline website). The change in tuition loans means that graduates attracted to the five year courses may now be propelled towards GEP courses, adding to the competition.

Other factors

Shorter courses may be attractive, offering the chance of less debt. However, some graduates fare better on an undergraduate course as they offer a lighter workload, different teaching styles, (slightly) less pressure, more holidays and the opportunity to continue earning some money. If you have dependents, a longer period of training may allow better pacing and balancing of responsibilities. Equally, speed may be of the essence. GEPs draw people from diverse backgrounds and ages, which will be a very different learning environment to an undergraduate course. For many, this is stimulating and positive, but not for others:

> *'I got through the pre-clinical but they were 18 difficult months as I didn't enjoy the mix in the group.'*

Summary

Whatever your starting point, carefully go through each prospectus, look at the websites, make a short-list and approach the admissions tutor directly if you are a non-standard entrant, as your four choices are irrevocable once submitted. Try to go to the open days and get a feel for the place.

If you are convinced medicine is truly your chosen path, then make sure you prepare well – be warned that this may take longer than you think. Be persistent, as many have testimonies of success on the second or third attempt.

> *'You have to ruthlessly organise your time and accept that some things in your life may well have to give. Hopefully that doesn't mean that the really important things, like your partner or your health, will suffer. But playing guitar in a rock band may well go the way of the dodo, and you know it's gone for good too.'*

> *'Every day I honestly feel it is such a privilege to be studying*

medicine, something I had dreamed of but thought could never be. Getting myself through the doors of the medical school as a mature student on an undergraduate course that first week was one of the hardest things I have ever done, but there has never been any regret. I think that if you are passionate about it, you can overcome difficulties and run with it, rather than live with regret.'

Key points:

- Consider the pros and cons of graduate entry programmes and undergraduate courses

- Before you apply, make sure you meet the academic requirements of your chosen medical schools

- Consider whether you need to take more A-levels or do an access course – if in doubt speak to an admissions tutor

- Plan ahead with loved ones as medical school can be stressful and will impact on your finances.

Useful websites

www.ucas.com
www.wanttobeadoctor.com
www.medschoolsonline.co.uk
www.newmediamedicine.com
www.study-medicine.co.uk
www.geocites.com/alexism1974/maturefaq
www.gamsatuk.org
www.ukcat.ac.uk
www.bmat.org.uk
www3.open.ac.uk/credit-transfer/index.htm
www.ukcisa.org.uk/student_fees_student_support.php

Chapter 7 Student finances

Dina Mansour

We are all familiar with the image of the stereotypical student holed up in a tiny grotty flat with scruffy clothes and only baked beans in the fridge. Whilst these students do exist, you don't need to be one of them. With careful planning, budgeting and maybe some part time work, all students should be able to live above the poverty line whilst at medical school.

A recent study, commissioned by the Sutton Trust, looked at the impact of financial considerations on 16–25 year olds' decisions on whether to participate in higher education. They reported that almost two thirds (59%) of 16–20 year olds who decided not to go on to Higher Education cited avoiding debt as a major factor in the decision. The BMA's medical student debt model projects that by the time new students filter through the five years of their course, an average medical student might owe the Student Loans Company (SLC) over £46,000 if they study in London and almost £37,000 if they study elsewhere. Medical students are hit with the same tuition fees and living costs as other students but also have the added expense of travelling between hospital sites and the university campus, buying expensive equipment and a long academic year. In addition, the course is usually at least two years longer than most other degrees. On the upside, there is a lot of financial help available and the financial rewards in the long run should outweigh your initial investment. Nevertheless, as a potential medical student, it is important that you appreciate the financial implications of your studies before embarking on your medical career.

Budgeting is the key to minimising debt and making your money go further. University will probably be the first chance you have had to manage your own finances. It is a good idea to sit down at the start of the academic year and work out how much you will receive from loans and grants and how much money you will need to spend on fees, accommodation and living costs. Scholarship-search.org.uk is a useful website that provides an online calculator which you can use to work out your income and expenditure over a year. With a bit of research, you should be able to find extra sources of funding as well as a multitude of student discounts and exemptions.

In this chapter we will take a closer look at the financial costs of going to medical school and the different sources of money available to you. We will also give you some tips on how to get the most out your time as a medical student without breaking the bank.

The costs

Funding your application
Even before reaching medical school you need to consider the cost of funding your application. The UKCAT entrance exam costs £60, while the BMAT costs £31 (see Chapter 3, prices correct in 2008). The GAMSAT exam for graduate entry will set you back £195. The cost of the BMAT and UKCAT can be reimbursed to candidates from the UK in receipt of full Education Maintenance Allowance (EMA), Job Seeker's Allowance or Income Support. More information on eligibility and on how to apply for the reimbursement bursaries can be found on the BMAT and UKCAT official websites. The costs of travelling

to interviews and of additional courses and books to help prepare for the application process also need to be taken into account.

Tuition fees

Tuition fees have added substantially to the cost of putting yourself through medical school. British students' contributions to tuition fees are means-tested. Depending on your parents' income you could have to pay up to £3,145 per year. The amount you have to pay is calculated by your local education authority (LEA), or the Students Awards Agency (SAAS) for those who live in Scotland. If you don't have parental support your tuition fee will depend on your own income.

From the fifth year of study onwards medical students are eligible for an NHS Bursary, which pays for tuition fees – this support is not means-tested and does not have to be repaid. This applies whether you do a five year or a six year course.

Up-to-date details of tuition fees, support and eligibility can be found in the student finance section of the government website www.direct.gov.uk.

Living costs

Rent constitutes the most substantial outgoing for any student moving away from home. The cost of renting accommodation depends on where you are studying (living in London, for example, is significantly more expensive than most other places) and whether you stay in student accommodation or rent privately. All medical schools offer accommodation, at least for the first year. The price (as well as the standard) varies from place to place, but it will generally be cheaper than renting privately, particularly as they tend to include all bills in the rent. An index of the average costs of both university and private accommodation can be found in the 'NUS accommodation costs survey', which is available online.

It can help to make a list of all the things that you will spend money on at university and try to estimate how much you will spend each week during term time. Here is an example based on the NUS accommodation costs survey (2006–7) and the Natwest student money matters survey (2005).

	Cost per week (£)	
Hall fees/Rent	81.80**	
Food	17.91*	Total cost (based on 42** week
Alcohol	17.09*	academic year)
Going out	14.75*	£212.44 × 42 = £8,922.48
Utility bills	12.71*	+ fees = £3,145.00 (2008–9)
Clothes/shoes	12.61*	Total (per year) £12,067.48
Transport	12.54*	
Eating out	11.85*	
Telephone bills	10.22*	
Books	9.25*	
Music	7.49*	
Laundry	4.22*	
Total	212.44	

** NUS accommodation costs survey 2006–7
* NatWest Student Money Matters Survey 2005

You will be exempt from paying council tax and a certificate of student exemption will be available from your university. There are special deals available for home insurance, mobile phones and travel (for example a young person's railcard) which can save you money. Several websites list all the latest student deals (for example www.students.com).

In-course costs

The cost of books, equipment and travel all adds up. If you're not careful, the cost of buying books can run into hundreds of pounds. You can minimise this expense through use of your university library, inheriting second hand books and buying used books at book fares or online. It is tempting to buy lots of new books at the start of each term in the hope that having the books will make you work harder. Think hard about which books you buy – it might be better to use the library at first and only buy the books you really need.

A decent stethoscope costs upwards of £55, but it is money well spent – for many people their first stethoscope will last throughout their career.

You might be entitled to help with travel costs incurred during training, such as to placements far away from your university. This help is usually means tested and comes from either your university or your LEA or SAAS.

Student memberships

In contrast to after you qualify, there are no obligatory membership payments as a medical student. You can sign up for medical indemnity (through the Medical Defence Union or the Medical Protection Society) but this is free and in fact both companies offer incentives to try to entice future doctors to sign up. These include free books, equipment, and discounts on courses and online examination practice sites. Some students also join the British Medical Association. Members receive a monthly international medical journal written specifically for students, which includes articles on wider issues affecting medical students, on electives and managing student debt for example. Subscription costs £39 per year.

Elective

The elective is a wonderful opportunity to travel and experience medicine in far-flung reaches of the world. However, this costs a lot of money. Most students who choose to travel abroad spend between £1,000–£2,000 for the two month trip, although many spend more. Each medical school provides a range of grants and many specialist organisations have awards available – see the website www.medicsworld.co.uk for a list.

Estimating your income

Student loan

Your LEA or SAAS will assess the amount of student loan available to you. Every medical student is eligible for at least 75 per cent of the full student loan, the remaining 25 per cent being means tested. Currently the maximum loan available is £4,625 (or £6,475 for students living in London). This amount rises with every additional week of study above the standard 30 week academic year. The interest rate on the student loan is in line with inflation and so the interest rate is much better than those offered by banks or other commercial loans. You will start repaying the loan as soon as your income reaches above £15,000 per year. You will then pay nine per cent of your income over £15,000 towards repaying your student loan. More information is available from the student loans company (www.slc.co.uk).

Grants and bursaries

Students from low income families and those having financial problems may be eligible for a hardship loan or grant. Hardship loans are added onto your student loan, while those who are still experiencing financial difficulties can apply for a hardship grant.

The NHS bursary pays for tuition fees in the fifth and sixth (for those who intercalate on a five year course) years of study. This is not means-tested. There is an additional maintenance component which is means-tested. This currently ranges from £1,936 to £5,064 (for a student living away from home in London). There are additional grants for older students and to cover childcare costs. These do not need to be repaid. However, students in receipt of an NHS bursary are no longer entitled to the full student loan. You will still be able to receive half the loan, which is, again, not means-tested.

Bank loans

Many high street banks offer loans for professional studies which are available to medical students, usually from the second year of study onwards. The amount available depends on the year of study and on what you plan to use the loan for. There are special loans available to help students pay for their elective. It is generally better to avoid any kind of bank loan as the interest rates can be crippling, but if you are unable to survive on the official student loan and additional money from grants and bursaries, it is worth shopping around to find which banks offer the best interest rates. Student bank accounts usually offer interest free overdrafts of up to £2,500 which can act as an important source of emergency cash.

Other sources of funding

For those who are well organised and have the time, there are a variety of sources of funding from a myriad of charities and trusts. Universities themselves often have a variety of obscure sources of funding that are not necessarily well advertised. The Royal colleges and other medical associations offer cash prizes for essay writing competitions, often publicised by medical schools. The closing dates for these competitions are spread throughout the year. Some medical schools will also have funds available to support projects in particular countries or in particular specialty areas. Other bursaries are more obscure: for example, some towns offer scholarships to students leaving to go to university, and there are special funds for children of airline pilots! If you are interested in joining the armed forces, they can provide sponsorship for your studies. These benefits include full tuition and fees, reimbursement for books and supplies, a monthly allowance, and 45 days of active duty each academic year for military training. Of course, you must serve on active duty after you graduate!

Many students use part time or holiday work to supplement money from loans and grants. This is more difficult at medical school because of the demanding nature of the course and the longer academic year. However the BMA's survey of medical students' finances shows that around a quarter of medical students work more than 16 hours per week during term time. Many take on part-time evening work during their pre-clinical years and spend at least part of their holidays temping, often as medical secretaries or health care assistants. Taking a summer job before starting the first year helps to tide you over until you first student loan instalment.

For many, parents play a crucial role in helping with finances: they offer loans at very competitive rates and even the odd bursary! However, students whose parents are not in a position to help financially should not feel that they cannot afford to go to medical school. Many grants are available exclusively to students from low income families. Universities are keen to encourage students from all socioeconomic groups to study medicine, and offer a range of hardship grants and bursaries.

The people at moneysavingexpert.com have come up with two mantras to keep students 'in the money', one for when you're hard-pressed for cash and one for when you aren't. They are definitely worth remembering!

FOR THOSE WHO ARE BROKE

Do I need it?
Can I afford it?
Have I checked if it's cheaper elsewhere?

FOR THOSE WHO AREN'T BROKE

Will I use it?
Is it worth it?
Have I checked if it's cheaper elsewhere?

If the answer to any of the questions is no, Don't Buy It.

Summary

Remember, your time as a student is meant to be enjoyed: it is the period in your life where you have the most freedom and least responsibility, and you should make the most of it. Medical school is designed to be accessible to all and a lack of money should not prevent you from applying. Nevertheless, without significant help from your family, you are likely to leave medical school with a sizable debt. It is therefore important to plan your finances. If you do this there is no reason why you can't fully enjoy your life as a medical student and reap the financial rewards of your investment throughout the remainder of your medical career.

Key points:

- Anyone should be able to afford to go to medical school, but being mindful of your finances will reduce the amount of debt you leave with.

- As a medical student your main outgoings will be fees, rent, travel, food, your elective, books, and equipment. It is a good idea to work out how much this is all going to cost so you know how much you have left for having fun!

- Good sources of income are student loans and grants, the NHS bursary and interest free overdrafts (for emergency cash). Avoid bank loans and other commercial loans if possible.

- If you do your research, you can find a variety of other sources of extra income and special student discounts to make your money go further.

Chapter 8 What do the early years of medical school involve?

Matthew Harrison

Once the dust of freshers' week has settled you will be expected to apply yourself fully to your medical studies. What you learn at medical school can be broken down into two parts; theory and practical, or often called pre-clinical and clinical teaching, (clinical being anything involving patients). Traditionally you spend the first two years of medical school learning the scientific basis of medicine and the remaining two years learning about patients and illness. Some medical schools retain this method of teaching but most now like to mix the two together to some degree. This chapter will deal with what you can expect in the first two years of medical school, still widely referred to as the pre-clinical years, you may have some clinical teaching early on but this will depend on where you go.

The core subjects that you study during these years are physiology, biochemistry, anatomy, pathology, pharmacology and molecular science.

Physiology and Biochemistry

Physiology is the study of the body's processes such as temperature regulation, pH regulation, breathing, metabolism, or anything that happens within the body. Biochemistry is how chemicals behave within the body – not like the organic chemistry you may have done at A Level but more similar to A-level biology; e.g. the Krebs cycle and the structure of body proteins such as haemoglobin.

Anatomy

Whereas physiology deals with how the body works, anatomy deals with what the body is; where the muscles, bones, nerves and blood vessels are in relation to one another. As you might expect, anatomy forms a large part of the early curriculum, as a good understanding of where everything is supposed to go is very important. Sometimes anatomy involves some embryology: where everything comes from in the developing embryo; this is helpful in understanding some quirks of the body.

Pathology

Pathology is the study of disease and disease processes, you might expect the study of disease to form the greatest part of medicine, but interestingly it often doesn't. You are mostly taught what everything is supposed to look like when it's normal before learning the diseases. As you progress through the course pathology will start to form an increasingly large part of the curriculum. At first, often just the study of pathological processes such as healing and cell death is taught, along with some basic histology (how things look under the microscope).

Pharmacology

Pharmacology is the study of drugs and their effects on the body. You will learn about how the body absorbs, excretes and deals with different types of chemicals and drugs, and what sorts of things can affect this process.

Molecular Science

This is an odd bunch of subjects, not taught enough of to justify having them as completely separate modules. They include things such as microbiology (bacteria), immunology (the immune system), oncology (cancer), and molecular genetics. Some of these aren't strictly molecular sciences but they have been included here for simplicity's sake.

As well as these purely science subjects, which form the reading, writing and arithmetic of your early studies, you will also be introduced to the more social and psychological side of medicine. These subjects include:

Interpersonal/Professional Development

This subject teaches you about how to be a good doctor; you learn communication skills and other important qualities surrounding the relationship between doctors and their patients. You may also receive a little tuition on medical law and ethics. This is hard to put into practise in the first couple of years but will give you an understanding of why doctors ask questions the way they do and hold you in good stead for when you transfer to the wards and see patients in the latter part of the course.

Epidemiology and Public Health

This subject deals with disease in the community, treating populations rather than individuals. Many courses teach you about research methods and statistics and how to read scientific papers in the context of public health.

During the first two years of medical school you will learn mainly about the theory behind medicine. However, there will be opportunities to start learning practical skills, which let's face it, is the fun bit.

CPR and Basic First Aid

In most places you will receive first aid training quite early on in the course. You will not be expected to attend and manage a cardiac arrest but you do need to have some skills to deal with basic problems.

Clinical Examination

How much of this you do will vary between medical schools, in most places you'll practise some very simple things, such as listening to a patient's heart or examining ears. The 'patients' will undoubtedly be your colleagues; although you may not see real patients it will give you an opportunity to be eased into examining patients before the third year comes along.

Now you know what you could expect to be taught when you first start at medical school, but exactly *how* will you be taught?

Teaching methods

How you will be taught varies between schools both in the structure and methods of teaching.

Traditional medical schools teach in a more 'subject-based' fashion. This means you have a course of anatomy, then a course of physiology, then a course of pharmacology all running separately alongside one another. Sometimes there may be some similarities between what you are being taught in each of them; say for instance if you're dissecting the heart in anatomy you might also be learning about the circulatory system in physiology, but this is not always the case.

Other medical schools rely more on the common themes between the subjects, this is a 'system-based' method of teaching. 'System-based' tuition teaches everything associated with a particular part of the body and then moves onto the next part. So in your first term you might be looking at the respiratory system, you are taught anatomy, physiology, pathology and everything else about this system. You then move onto the next part of the body, learn everything to do with that, and so on until you have covered the whole body. There are obviously pros and cons to both of these methods and both lend themselves to different styles of teaching.

'Subject-based' courses are more likely to involve much more didactic teaching. This is the type of teaching you will probably be used to from school, where you sit and listen to somebody else talking, make notes and try to absorb information. 'System-based' courses can be taught didactically but more often they involve PBL-like teaching.

Practically speaking either 'subject' or 'system' based teaching will expose you to a range of teaching methods:

Lectures

If you are on a medical course other than one that is PBL-based then you are likely to spend a great deal of your time in the lecture theatre. Lectures are the most efficient way to teach a large number of students. Most of your lectures will take place with your entire year and sometimes there may even be students from other courses like Dentistry, Pharmacology or Neuroscience. You may end up with a couple of hundred students in the theatre. Your task in lectures is to sit, listen and learn. In some cases this is not easy, in other cases the lecture will be excellent and you will acquire all the information you need. Lectures usually last between 45 minutes and an hour.

Tutorials/Seminars

These are the mainstay of the PBL course although most medical courses make use of them. In a tutorial there will be a small group of students, usually around ten, and a facilitator or group co-ordinator who will be a member of the teaching staff.

In PBL you will work with this group for most of your teaching, sharing tasks that arise from problems and bringing them back to the group. An advantage of tutorials is that they allow discussion, which is impossible in a lecture theatre. Because of this, even in non-PBL courses tutorials are often used to teach things like communication skills, professional development and medical ethics – subjects that can arouse a great deal of debate. As tutorials are less intense than lectures they may last longer – perhaps around two hours.

Practicals

As you go through the subject areas in medical school, there will be practical sessions that aim to give you a better understanding of them and help those who do not learn well from lectures. Topics such as histology can't easily be taught in lecture format and you really need to adopt a hands-on approach to understand it. Hence practical teaching can involve anything from analysing the expiratory gases of your colleagues to examining gut epithelia under the microscope. Practical sessions may require you to write up what you have done or work through a set of questions before the session.

If you go to a medical school that uses dissection to teach anatomy you can look forward to many hours in the dissection room. Dissection sessions run in a similar way to tutorials: usually a small group of you will share a cadaver (dead body) and over a period of time you will work through tasks, gradually dissecting the entire body. Dissection is a great way to learn anatomy. If you are lucky enough to do it you may find it daunting but ultimately very rewarding. If you don't want to dissect then don't despair. Anatomy can still be taught very well using prosections, which are bits of cadavers that have already been dissected and fixed. Newer methods such as computer models are equally fascinating and probably just as effective. Dissections and practical sessions last much longer than lectures or tutorials and usually take up half a day, but some may last all day. Some practicals may last all day if you have to take multiple measurements or the drugs that you have administered to a colleague take some time to take effect.

Clinical Skills Sessions

Clinical skills sessions, like practical sessions, are hands on and lots of fun. These sessions usually comprise of groups of students being taught a particular skill such as how to examine the lungs. You learn invasive procedures (e.g. taking blood) on models and when you feel confident with these, you can practise on real patients.

Placements

Placements do not form a large part of your teaching early on as they are more for the clinical years. However, you may have some short early placements such as visiting a GP's surgery or a hospital once a month. These placements give you the opportunity to practise some of the things you have learnt in your communication or clinical skills sessions.

They also give you a taste of what medicine is like outside of the lecture theatre.

Exams

Some of the exams at medical school will be in formats that you are already familiar with: essays, short written answers or multiple choice questions. There are also some new exam formats you will be less familiar with:

True/False/Abstain (TFA)

Sitting TFA exams is a skill in itself, which you will soon pick up if you are at a medical school that uses them. In these exams you are presented with a set of statements which, as the name suggests, will either be true or false. The difference comes in the marking: if you answer a question correctly you score one point, but if you answer a question incorrectly you score minus one point. If you choose to abstain and not answer that question you score zero. So say in a set of five questions you answer three correctly, one incorrectly and abstain on one question, you would score two out of five.

Spotters

These are most commonly used in anatomy, but can also be used to test other subject areas such as histology and pharmacology. In a spotter there will be a number of stations that you move around every few minutes when a bell rings. At each station there will be an item, usually a prosection, bone, x-ray, or picture. It may have a label on it, an arrow, or nothing at all. Associated with each station will be one or two questions, the first question is usually something like 'what is this structure?' or 'what is the structure labelled 'A'?' The second question is usually something to do with the thing you have just identified, for example, 'what does it do?' or 'by what artery is it supplied?' You will need to write the answer on your paper and move on to the next station when you hear the bell.

Vivas

Vivas are spoken exams, similar to interviews. You sit before a person or persons and discuss a topic or a report that you have produced. The examiners will ask you questions to gauge your understanding of the topic and score you appropriately.

Intercalation

Intercalation was mentioned in Chapter 3 as being an important factor to consider when deciding which medical school to apply to. But what exactly is it and what does it mean for your studies? Some medical courses give you the opportunity to study another degree as part of your medical training; this is called an intercalated degree. At some universities, such as Oxford or Cambridge, an intercalated BSc is compulsory. At most medical schools it is optional, and only a minority can take one. At Nottingham the intercalated degree is an integral part of the course.

What sort of things can you study?

In most places the intercalated degree is strongly medically-related. In other places, usually where the degree is optional, there is much more choice, although most options are science-based subjects such as physiology genetics or psychology. There are some non-science degrees around: for example, select universities are now offering degrees in clinical management and ethics.

To intercalate, or not to intercalate?

Pros

- You leave medical school with another degree.

- You learn skills that other medical students may not have, such as learning to read and critique scientific papers, juggling statistics or even more practical tasks, for example, culturing bacteria or analysing DNA on electrophoresis gels. Skills like this may give you an advantage in a competitive specialty.

- You will have the opportunity to participate in research and having your name in print. An intercalated degree can set you up for a career in academic medicine.

- If you decide that medical school is not for you or you have to leave for some other reason, you will have that degree to take with you, and your time at medical school won't have been entirely wasted.

Cons

- The major con of course is the extra work involved, and don't forget the extra exams!
- Much of the work, especially if the degree is a medical science subject, is very 'sciencey', and often of little clinical relevance. Some of what you learn you may never use again unless you go on to do research in that field.
- In most places taking an intercalated degree means adding an extra year onto your studies; this is usually added between your second and third year.

Key points:

- Medical teaching was traditionally divided into pre-clinical and clinical teaching. Some places retain this system but most now have at least a partially mixed course.

- Your first couple of years in medical school will be mainly spent learning the basic sciences.

- The majority of teaching will be via lectures if you are on a more traditional course or tutorials if you are on a PBL course.

- Unfortunately you will have exams – these will come in a variety of formats.

- An intercalated degree may be offered as part of the course and although it involves more work, it is a good way to learn new skills.

Chapter 9 Reaching your goal – what do the final years of medical school involve?

Tom Nolan

Introduction

The final years of medical school are challenging and the learning curve is steep, but for most they are also the most enjoyable and rewarding as you begin to see what being a doctor is really like. By the time you reach your third year you will have spent some time in hospital and will be familiar with the ward environment. From now on though you will be based at hospitals and general practices and taught by specialists, junior doctors and patients.

The final years of medical school are often referred to as the clinical years, although this distinction is less true now than it was in the past. The structure of these years varies between medical schools (see Table 1). Most, however, begin with a short introductory course which is followed by clinical rotations, or firms. During each rotation you and several other students are attached to a specialty within a hospital or general practice. The first clinical year tends to cover general medicine and its specialties. The second year might cover things like paediatrics, psychiatry and obstetrics and gynaecology. The final year is focused on preparing you for starting work as a junior doctor – and your final exams! For many, the highlight of these three years is the elective period – an opportunity to study medicine anywhere in the world.

Table 1. Clinical course structure at three UK medical schools.

	Brighton & Sussex Medical School	Newcastle University Medical School	Royal Free & University College Medical School
Year 3	Introductory clinical knowledge & skills course. Eight week rotations in medicine, surgery, obstetrics and gynaecology, paediatrics, mental health and elderly care. Scientific basis of medicine course and student selected modules run throughout the year.	Introductory clinical knowledge & skills course. Rotations in Reproductive and child health, chronic illness, disability and rehabilitation, mental health, public health and infectious diseases. Half a day each week in general practice.	Introductory clinical knowledge & skills course. Four rotations: general medical specialties; general medicine and medicine in the community; surgery and anaesthetics; care of the older person/ orthopaedics and rheumatology.
Year 4	Musculoskeletal medicine and surgery; oncology; haematology & palliative care; neurology & neurosurgery; dermatology; ophthalmology/ENT; infectious diseases. Elective. Individual research project.	12-week course in clinical sciences and investigative medicine. 30-week period of student-selected components and elective study. Elective.	Women's health and communicable diseases, psychiatry and neurology with ophthalmology, and child and family health with dermatology.
Year 5	Regional attachments, rotating through major specialties. 1 week emergency medicine attachment. Preparation for clinical practice course runs throughout the year.	Regional attachments in primary and community care, women's and children's care, mental health care. Preparation for practice and hospital-based practice. Shadowing course after final exams.	Regional attachments in medicine and surgery, Emergency medicine. General practice and oncology. Elective. Student Selected Components (SSCs).

Getting used to patients

How do you approach a complete stranger who is sick in hospital, who might be struggling to breathe or have terminal cancer, and ask them to talk to you about their illness? What do you ask? How long should you talk to them for? How are you going to examine them if every movement they make causes them pain? Being a medical student isn't easy! Fortunately, the overwhelming majority of patients are incredibly friendly and willing to be questioned, prodded and poked. In fact, many find it helpful to talk to someone about their illness. You'll be doing this on an almost daily basis as you learn how to clerk patients – that is, take a history from and examine them.

Taking a history

History taking is probably the most useful and most overlooked skill that doctors learn. Experts can tease out all the information they need from a patient within minutes, and make them feel that they have been listened to and cared for at the same time. To get to this stage takes lots of practise and a great deal of hard work and reflection – it's no wonder that many doctors never really master it.

What is a history? It's really an account of everything about a patient that might be relevant to their health. When you think about it, almost anything can be, so it can take a long time to find all this out! There are physical, psychological, genetic, social, economic, geographic, and many more factors that can contribute to illness. By putting all of these things together, doctors are able to work out how best to help their patients.

Taking a history can be daunting. In many ways, though, it's not much different to trying to find out some gossip from a friend – the questions you ask may be very similar: what happened? Who saw you? Has it happened before? What were you thinking? How do you feel now? Do you think it will happen again? All of these questions could be asked to an elderly lady who has had a fall. You could just as easily ask them to your best friend if you'd just found out they'd been caught behind the bike sheds with someone from school!

Once you've found out all this information – about the patient, not your friend, that is – how do you relay it back to someone in a logical order that is easy to understand? The standard way of ordering a history is as follows:

Presenting complaint
This is what made the patient seek medical advice.

History of presenting complaint
A posh way of saying what happened. It can be hard to take a patient's story and turn it into a concise and relevant summary that others can follow.

Past medical history
It's important to know what medical problems patients have had in the past. For instance, a man who has high blood pressure is more likely have a heart attack than someone who does not have high blood pressure.

Drug history
There are thousands of drugs around – and they all have side effects. Finding out from a patient what they take every day can be quite a challenge!

Family history
This can be crucial in determining if someone is at risk of getting a disease, e.g. breast cancer.

Personal history

What does the patient think is wrong? What ideas do they have about their symptoms? What do they want from their doctor? Answering these questions can be the key to tackling illness and can make the difference between a satisfied patient and an angry one. Overlook them at your peril!

Social history

Drinking, smoking, drugs, take-aways and anything else that you were ever told you shouldn't do!

Systems review

To round up and make sure that no stone has been left unturned, a top to toe review of all symptoms.

Students in their clinical years might take several histories each week. This can take a long time, especially at first. Writing them up and reading about the symptoms, diseases and medications is also time consuming. However, this is still the best way to learn, as talking to someone with a disease really brings it to life and makes it memorable.

The clinical examination: using your stethoscope

The stethoscope is the great symbol of the medical profession. Read any medical textbook or go to any website about medicine and you're almost guaranteed to see one somewhere. In a modern hospital with no white coats or ties they can be the only clue that a person is a doctor. It can be argued that their practical value is not as great as it once was, with the increased availability of scans and blood tests. Nevertheless, learning to use a stethoscope and perform a full examination is still a key part of the undergraduate medical curriculum, and is an essential skill for any junior doctor.

Most medical schools begin the first clinical year with an introductory course. Much of this is devoted to learning the main examinations (cardiovascular, respiratory, abdominal, neurological and locomotor). You may be taught by final year medical students or junior doctors, which makes it a more informal and fun way to start your clinical studies.

Practical skills

A big part of life as a junior doctor is having to take blood, insert cannulas (plastic tubes to give intra-venous fluids through) and other bits of plastic like catheters and drains. They can be difficult at first but once you get the hang of them, they can be really satisfying to do. You'll learn how to do these things on plastic models first, then under supervision on patients.

Communication skills

Teaching in communication skills begins in the first year of medical school and continues throughout the clinical years.

When you start seeing patients it can be hard to work out what it was that they came to see you about. Imagine you are a GP and a patient comes to see you about back pain. You might start asking them about where the pain is, when it started, how severe it is and so on. You may be satisfied that the pain isn't that bad and has no serious cause and send them home with some pain killers. You might even wonder why they bothered to come to see you about such a minor problem! Communication skills teaching encourages you to look at things differently: what was the patient hoping you would do for them? Did they want some pain killers or just some reassurance? Or are they depressed or having troubles at work? What are they worried about? What do they think has caused it? Asking these sorts of questions is often more useful than just focusing on symptoms.

Communication skills teaching also covers different styles of consultation, dealing with angry patients, breaking bad news, and communicating with colleagues. Much of the teaching is in small groups, often in a communication skills suite with cameras and one way glass so you can watch each other and give feedback.

Ethics and law

It is impossible to practise medicine without having to make ethical decisions. Admittedly, 'who do you give the organ to?' scenarios that are popular with interviewers don't occur every day, but others do. It might be that a confused patient is refusing treatment, or a nurse asking for sleeping tablets for a noisy patient who is keeping the rest of the ward awake. A concerned mother might ask you to disclose information about her 15-year-old daughter's contraception. Or you might need to decide whether an elderly patient should be resuscitated if they have a cardiac arrest. Having to make these decisions can be extremely stressful and the consequences of making a bad decision could be disastrous – both for you and the patient. Your ethics teaching at medical school gives you a really useful basis to help you make these decisions as a doctor.

Specialties

During your clinical years, you are taken on a whistle-stop tour of medicine. This is a really great opportunity to sample the large variety of subjects within medicine, from the excitement and stress of emergency medicine to the more strategic field of public health. Everyone is different and different things appeal to different people. Nobody should expect to enjoy everything. However, it's a good idea to try to get as involved as possible in each firm as it may be your only opportunity to sample these specialties before you have to decide what to specialise in (see Chapter 10).

The main specialties covered during your clinical years are as follows:

Medicine

More time is spent on medical firms than any of the others – that's because there's a lot to cover. Firms include cardiology, endocrinology, gastroenterology, infectious diseases, neurology, respiratory medicine and rheumatology.

Surgery

There's a real contrast between medicine and surgery. Going from one firm to the other can be refreshing and challenging. Your time is divided between the wards, out-patient clinics and the operating theatre. In theatre you get the opportunity to assist in operations, cutting, suturing and more often than not holding instruments for hours on end. The two major areas are general surgery (things like hernia, bowel and appendix operations) and orthopaedics (hammering nails into bones). You will also get to sample other specialties such as vascular surgery, neurosurgery, plastics, ENT and maxillofacial surgery.

Obstetrics and Gynaecology

It's a great privilege to be present at the birth of a child and is an experience that few medical students forget. It's not everyone's cup of tea, of course, so if this is the sort of thing that you think you might not like (and it can be pretty messy!) don't worry. However, having pre-conceived ideas about it can be damaging. By launching into things you can overcome your fears and anxieties and often be surprised by how enjoyable you find them.

Paediatrics

'Paeds' – as almost everyone calls it – covers all ages from birth to teenagers. As such, it is a very diverse field with a lot of variety. During this rotation you will spend time at a neonatal unit and learn how to assess a sick child.

Psychiatry

From high security mental health units to child and adolescent psychiatry and psychotherapy, you are bound to come across some fascinating stories and behaviour. Taking a history from a patient with a mental illness is very difficult, both for you and the patient. Mental illness is very common and anyone considering a career as a GP will need to know a lot about it.

General Practice

Almost half of medical students will become GPs. However, ask a group of them what they want to specialise in, and few will say General Practice. This specialty is often looked down on by students, many of whom find it less exciting than hospital medicine and too 'touchy feely'. In actual fact, being a GP is extremely challenging, both in terms of the breadth of knowledge required and the need for good communication skills. During this placement you will spend time watching experienced GPs with patients and the chance to see patients by yourself.

On-call experience

During each rotation you will have the opportunity to experience front line medicine during on-calls. The on-call team of doctors sees all the new admissions to hospital under their specialty. This is the best place to see interesting things (like chest drains, lumbar punctures and emergency operations) and learn the art of making a diagnosis. You will often get to see patients before the doctors do, which can be really exciting – and it prevents you from peeking at the notes to find out what the diagnosis is.

Student Selected Components (SSCs)

All medical schools are required to include SSCs as part of their course. SSCs are a chance to spend time learning about topics that are of particular interest to you. They can be about clinical topics or research or humanities based. Examples of student selected components include international health, teaching medical students, medical journalism and forensic pathology. Part of the purpose of them is to encourage you to be self-directed in your learning, so the more you put in, the more you're likely to get out of them.

Elective

During your final two years you will have the chance to go on an elective. This is an opportunity to experience medicine in a different environment, almost anywhere in the world. Some students decide to go to a developing country, while others may wish to go to a centre of excellence in the USA or Asia. Many go to Australia to experience medicine on a beach whilst others stay in the UK, perhaps doing a research project.

Experiencing medicine in a developing country or in a completely different culture is a truly memorable experience. Being in such a different environment with different people and seeing diseases that you've never seen before – or even heard of – can be overwhelming. But if you plan your trip well and do lots of research before you go so you know what to expect, you should have a great time.

Final year – preparing for practice

The final year of medical school is designed to get you ready for life as a junior doctor. You'll return to general medicine and surgery to sharpen up your clinical skills as you start to buckle down and revise for finals. These placements are usually away from the main teaching hospitals. You might have to live in hospital accommodation as the distances to travel from home can be great. Hospital accommodation has a variable reputation to say the least, but it is improving. Living with a bunch of other students somewhere new is actually, as you might imagine, a lot of fun.

Exams and Finals

The dreaded exams! The gateway to becoming a doctor, and the most disliked part of medical school. Like it or not, though, you're going to have to pass them if you want to get those all important letters after your name.

Your exams in the first two clinical years will cover the rotations you have just been on. These may be written exams and/ or OSCEs (see below).

Unlike the United States, where there is a single exit exam for all medical students, each medical school in the UK sets their own exams. As a result the methods of assessment vary, but the most widely used are OSCEs, OSLERS and written exams.

OSCEs

OSCE stands for Observed Structured Clinical Examination. Essentially, an OSCE is a series of short practical stations where you demonstrate your doctorly skills. Each station is different – one might be to examine somebody's neck, whilst the next one might be to take blood from a plastic arm. You are scored against a mark scheme to ensure that everyone is treated fairly. OSCEs have replaced the traditional 'short case' practical exam which was far less structured and which many felt were unfair (the lack of a specific mark scheme meant that the examiner could pass or fail someone on a whim).

OSLERs

An Objective Structured Long Examination Record (OSLER) is a standardised method of rating clerkings that covers history taking, examination skills and your approach to diagnosis and management.

Written exams

Most written exams are multiple choice exams. There are several types of these including True/False, Single Best Answer (SBA) and Extended Matching Questions (EMQ). SBAs ask you to pick the most appropriate option from a list of possible answers. EMQs typically give a long list of possible answers and ask you to select from the list the correct answers to a series of questions. These types of questions test your ability to apply what you know to specific problems.

Portfolios

Some people try to avoid putting the hours in on the wards and get through medical school by just cramming for exams. To discourage this, your medical school will ask you to keep a portfolio or logbook of all the things you've seen and done during your clinical attachments. If you can't show that you've been busy, you may have to repeat an attachment or even a whole year.

Summary

Most students really enjoy their clinical years. Moving from the lecture theatre or tutorial room to the ward is a welcome change of scene. Being part of a firm of several students, you explore medicine together and make lots of new friends. As you get more confident in your abilities, you begin to understand more about medicine and feel more able to tackle the challenges that it throws up. With such a lot of topics to cover in just three years, the time goes by very quickly and before you know it, you'll be getting ready to start work as a doctor.

Key points

- During the clinical years you learn how to clerk patients – take a history, examine them and make a management plan.

- You rotate through all the major specialties and learn practical skills, communication skills, ethics and law.

- During your elective you have the opportunity to experience medicine anywhere in the world. Plan it carefully and you'll have a great experience.

- You will be assessed throughout your clinical years with practical and written assessments.

- Finals are the most feared part of medical school but most people get through them unscathed!

Chapter 10 Career paths and choosing a specialty

Tom Nolan

Introduction

Medicine is diverse. Depending on what specialty you choose you could spend your career doing ward rounds, in the operating theatre, in a clinic, behind a microscope or even at a desk. Deciding which specialty to train for and dedicate your career to can be really hard. You might be happy just to choose your favorite, but other factors like hours, pay, flexibility and competitiveness can also influence your decision.

Specialty training in the UK is undergoing a radical overhaul, causing great controversy and unrest amongst doctors. The new training system, called Modernising Medical Careers (MMC) aims to improve the quality of medical education and make the career paths of doctors more efficient. Many changes, such as Specialty Training and the Foundation Programme have already been introduced. Other changes, such as to the role of the Consultant, have yet to be confirmed. This chapter delves into the history of MMC, describes the career path of a doctor in the UK and offers some advice on how to choose the right specialty for you.

Modernising Medical Careers

Modernising Medical Careers (MMC) was launched in February 2003. It was introduced for two main reasons: to increase the amount of care provided by fully trained specialists and to improve training by introducing a detailed curriculum, competency assessments and better supervision of trainees. With many doctors unhappy with the new system, it's worth considering what was wrong with the old one.

The NHS Plan

The NHS Plan, published in 2000 by the then recently elected Labour government, described the NHS as a 1940s system operating in a 21st century world. According to the plan, there were 'too few doctors and nurses and other key staff to carry out all the treatments required.' As a result it aimed to create 7,500 more Consultants and 2,000 more GPs. It wasn't clear at the time how the government planned to do this: 1,000 more places at medical school were promised, but it would be at least ten years before any of these doctors would be fully trained. In any case, the main purpose of creating more medical school places was to reduce the reliance on doctors trained abroad. So where were all these Consultants and GPs going to come from? The answer to this question lies in the structure of the old training system.

The old system (see Figure 1) of pre-registration house officers (PRHOs), senior house officers (SHOs) and specialist Registrars (SpRs), which had existed for decades, was loved for its flexibility but created a lot of problems at SHO level. After passing finals you would be thrown in at the deep end, with little advice or support into a 'sink or swim' environment. After a year you would become an SHO, a sort of desert island where you could live in relative comfort for as long as you liked. Once you'd built up enough experience and energy, you could swim onwards towards any specialty of your choosing provided you had the correct documentation (in the form of the relevant post-graduate qualification such as the MRCP for general medicine and a Registrar 'number'). Many would get stuck at SHO level, being unable to get a 'number' (since these were strictly limited by the number of Consultant posts) whilst others were happy to stay as an SHO, gaining greater experience and without the responsibilities of being a specialist Registrar.

Unfinished business

After the NHS Plan, the SHO position was scrutinised by Sir Liam Donaldson, the Chief Medical Officer (the most senior advisor to the government on health). His report, 'Unfinished Business', published in September 2002, signaled the beginning of the end of the SHO grade. It criticised the stand alone nature of over half of the posts, which forced SHOs to apply for new jobs every six months. It highlighted the lack of career guidance and the wide range in the quality of SHOs. The need to pass tough exams before becoming an SpR was leading to many SHOs not progressing as quickly as they would like, making the grade feel more like a detention camp than a desert island.

Perhaps the most significant part of Unfinished Business, however, was its advice regarding the Consultant grade. It argued that by the time doctors reach the level of Consultant, most are more specialised than they need to be to provide the services that the NHS needs. A more focused and structured junior doctor training programme was required to 'produce fully-trained specialists with . . . skills more closely attuned to the current needs of the NHS'.

And so, the following year, MMC was launched. The first stage of the new career path, the Foundation Programme, launched in 2005. The next stage, Specialty Training was implemented in 2007 with the infamous Medical Training Application System (MTAS – see below). The first doctors to achieve the end point of their training, the Certificate of Completion of Training

(CCT), will begin to come through in the next couple of years. The exact role of doctors who have attained their CCT remains to be seen (see Becoming a Consultant, below).

The Foundation Programme

The aim of the Foundation Programme is to form a stepping stone between medical school and specialty training – it's a big step up, so that can only be a good thing! It's much more structured than the old pre-registration house officer (PRHO) year. For instance, you must complete various assessments and you have a supervisor who sets objectives with you and monitors your progress.

During this time, various clinical and non-clinical skills (or 'competencies') are assessed. This is done using four types of assessment: DOPS, mini-CEX, CBDs and mini-ePATs.

DOPS stands for Directly Observed Procedural Skills. Examples include taking blood or inserting a catheter. A senior doctor will watch you and score you against certain criteria.

A **mini-CEX** is a mini-Clinical Evaluation Exercise. It assesses doctor-patient interactions. Examples include taking a history or giving some bad news to a patient. Again, this is done on the ward with one of your seniors.

CBDs, or Case Based Discussions, involve presenting a case and answering questions about the diagnosis and management.

A **mini-ePAT**, or 360 degree assessment, looks at how well those who work with you think you're doing. They rate your ability across a range of skills including communication, timekeeping and attitude.

Each foundation year (FY1 and FY2) is divided into three or four blocks, known as 'firms'. FY1 jobs range from general

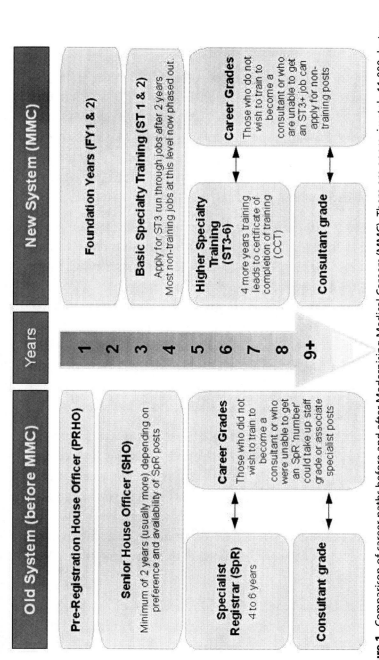

Figure 1. Comparison of career paths before and after Modernising Medical Careers (MMC). There are approximately 11,000 doctors altogether in foundation years 1 and 2, 30,000 in basic specialty training and 10,000 in higher specialty training. There are 37,000 Consultants and 40,000 GPs. The diagram above is based on careers in general medicine – other specialties vary: Paediatrics training is currently eight years long and trainees do not need to reapply after two years; General Practice specialty training is only three years long – the third year (ST3) is known as the GP Registrar year.

medicine or surgery to ENT or renal medicine. FY2 jobs can also include A&E and general practice.

On a day-to-day level, the job of a foundation year trainee is very similar to that of the old PRHO or SHO. FY1 doctors do many of the basic tasks that keep the firm ticking over. Most days start with a ward round, usually with a Registrar or Consultant. Your job is to know where all the patients are, write in their notes, and make a list of all the things that need doing for each patient that day – and then do them.

For many, the most terrifying thing about starting the job is carrying a 'bleep'. Most bleeps are about mundane things, like a nurse wanting fluids or pain killers prescribing. Every now and then, though, bleeps are for urgent matters. According to your disposition, this is the part of the job that you either love or hate – but remember, hating it doesn't mean you're a bad doctor! Either way, one of the great things about the Foundation Programme is that by the end of it everyone will have received training in Advanced Life Support (ALS), making assessing and treating sick patients much less stressful.

On-call duties vary from job to job. In some you work a standard day, beginning at 8 or 9 o'clock each morning, and leaving at 5pm with an evening on-call about once a week, and a weekend on-call every few weeks. New limits to working hours mean that from 2009 the maximum working week must be 48 hours. As a result, lots of jobs are changing to a shift system, with fewer days at work but longer or more irregular hours whilst there.

Most Foundation Year 2 (FY2) jobs are part of a rota shared with doctors in the first years of Specialty Training. All FY2s are required to spend at least four months working in acute medicine – usually A&E or on a Medical Assessment Unit.

Specialty Training

From August 2007, all SHO and SpR jobs were combined to form the new Specialty Registrar (StR) grade. It was originally intended that anyone who had an StR job would be guaranteed a job until they had completed their training. That was good news for a lot of doctors, because it meant they wouldn't have to apply for new jobs every six months like they used to.

Soon after this system was introduced, two big problems emerged. Firstly, the centralised application system, MTAS (Medical Training Application Service), was dogged by technical problems and security scares. The second problem was associated with guaranteeing a job until training was complete (which could be up to eight years). Although this was good for those who got on the training schemes, it wasn't such good news for anyone who didn't. If you didn't get an StR job you would have to take a non-training job and would have very little chance of getting an StR job later. In some specialties the number of StR training posts available was dwarfed by the numbers of doctors applying for them. For example, in the London deanery in 2007, there were over 22 applicants for each radiology training post. Competition for jobs was fierce throughout the country, with three or more applications per job in the majority of cases. Many doctors were faced with the prospect of having no training job at all. Hundreds of doctors had to ask themselves some really hard questions: were they happy to work for the rest of their careers in a non-Consultant role? Should they pick a less popular specialty? Should they move abroad or even leave medicine altogether? This, taken with most doctors' view that their applications were not being fairly considered using MTAS, led to great unrest amongst doctors and a growing feeling that the profession was in crisis.

MTAS was scrapped and the selection process for 2008 was

reviewed. An independent inquiry into MMC, led by Professor Sir John Tooke, recommended sweeping changes to post-graduate medical training. Most training jobs have been 'uncoupled', so that after completing Core Training (ST1 and ST2), trainees must re-apply for jobs in higher Specialty Training (the major exceptions are General Practice and Paediatrics). Most non-training jobs at ST1 and ST2 level have been turned into training jobs. It is expected that in uncoupled specialties there will be far more posts in ST1 and ST2 than in ST3 and above. The bottleneck of SHOs wishing to become Registrars that MMC aimed to make disappear will probably still exist.

Becoming a Consultant

There is a great deal of debate about what it will mean to be a Consultant in the future. Many fear that as a result of MMC a new grade of doctor, dubbed the 'sub-Consultant', will be created. These doctors would be responsible for most ward and out-patient work and would refer rare or more complex things to '-ologists', a more senior version of the old fashioned Consultant. This is alluded to in Unfinished Business:

> 'such a model would work best if at the point of completion of the shorter first phase period of higher specialist training, the doctor was eligible for a Consultant level post in their chosen specialty. So they would become a Consultant in for example: general internal medicine or general paediatrics. This would make a distinction between two categories of specialist: the "generalist" Consultant and what some have dubbed the "ologists" '

In other words, most of the 7,500 new Consultants promised in the NHS Plan are likely to be general Consultants, with fewer, more specialised doctors to look after the most complex patients.

Choosing a specialty

One consequence of MMC is that doctors have to decide earlier what they want to specialise in. Some people you meet seem to have known what they wanted to do since before they could walk – they're usually surgeons! Most aren't so certain and will change their minds several times before finally deciding. There are 54 specialties within the NHS so it's little wonder that it's so difficult to make up your mind (for those who are curious the smallest specialty is sport and exercise medicine with only four Consultants, whilst the biggest is general practice with over 36,000). With such a range of options, it's definitely worth making the most of the opportunities at medical school to sample different kinds of medicine. After you qualify, you will have 18 months working as a doctor before you have to make up your mind. This isn't enough time to try everything, so it's all the more important to think about it as a student.

How to choose

What type of person are you? Do you like excitement and drama or do you like the quieter life? Do you love to talk and be around lots of different people or are you happier doing things on your own or in a small team? Do you love to be in charge and have responsibilities or are you more of a team player? Are you the sort of person who likes time to consider things before doing them or do you prefer to 'just get on with it' and deal with the consequences later? You will ask yourself many of these questions (and many more) when considering whether medicine is the right career for you (see Chapter 2). They are also relevant when choosing your specialty. Thinking about these things and talking to others about them can really help you to make the right decision.

Some specialties have a lot of emergencies where you need to make life and death decisions very quickly – examples include Obstetrics, General Surgery and Emergency Medicine. Others, such as Public Health, Histopathology and General Practice allow you to consider things for a while before reaching decisions. Other factors to consider are:

Hours – including number of hours worked and how often – if ever – you have to work weekends or at night.

Competition for places – This varies greatly between specialties. Information about numbers of posts and applicants for them is available on the MMC website.

Pay and private practice – Pay for Consultants is higher than for career grade doctors and some specialties have more opportunities to work in the private sector than others.

Patient contact – As you progress up the ladder, the time spent with patients reduces and the time spent doing paperwork increases. Those wanting to stay 'on the shop floor' and avoid desk work might consider career grade jobs or general medicine.

Flexibility – General practice is well known for its flexibility – many GPs choose to work fewer hours to allow them more time with their family and pursue other interests.

Research – If you fancy being the next Alexander Fleming there are academic training options in most specialties. These allow you to split your time between clinical practice and research.

Many medical schools and hospital trusts have careers services that can offer valuable advice. Sci59 is a computer program that asks you 59 questions about you and suggests which specialties are most suited to you. Another excellent source of advice are your teachers and Consultants. During medical school you meet dozens of doctors. Try to imagine yourself doing their job – can you see yourself in their shoes? If there is a teacher or doctor at medical school who you look up to or build a rapport with, why not ask them to talk to you about your options? Ask them how they got to where they are and what things you can do to improve your chances of reaching a similar position. Most will be more than happy to help and might even ask you to help them with an audit or some research.

Once you've made up your mind, think about how you can build your CV to maximise your chances of getting the job. In fact, even if you're still not sure what to do, it's still worth becoming involved in some projects – the application system currently being used awards points for things like presentations, publications and prizes. These are the things that can set you apart from the rest of the crowd and help you to get your dream job.

Changing your mind
Most doctors admit to changing their minds several times before finally deciding on what they want to do. If you change your mind after you start specialty training, it's not the end of the world – you can apply to begin specialty training in another field. Your interviewers will be curious as to why you changed your mind, but they shouldn't count it against you if you can show that you're really committed to your new specialty.

Summary
The upheaval of introducing a new career structure in the form of MMC has caused great distress to doctors. As worrying as all this change can be, it is important to keep a sense of

perspective. Medicine has always been competitive. The investment in training and education by the government *has* increased the numbers of jobs available and therefore increased opportunities. Working hours are shorter and although this has implications for training, efforts are being made to make sure that training does not suffer. With hard work and dedication it is still possible for doctors to reach their goals provided they think carefully about their careers and choose the right specialty for them.

Key points:

- Modernising Medical Careers (MMC) was introduced to improve standards and increase the share of patients being treated by fully trained specialists.

- Newly qualified doctors enter the two year Foundation Programme, which aims to train doctors in basic skills and give them a broad introduction to medicine.

- Specialty Training consists of basic and higher Specialty Training. At the end of their training doctors achieve a Certificate of Completion of Training (CCT), which allows them to apply for Consultant or general practice jobs.

- You have less than two years as a doctor before you have to decide what to specialise in – start thinking about it early!

- Think about what you can do to enhance your CV to increase your chances of getting the job you want.

Useful websites

The NHS Plan
http://www.dh.gov.uk/en/Publicationsandstatistics/Publica-
tions/PublicationsPolicyAndGuidance/DH_4010198

Unfinished business – Sir Liam Donaldson, CMO
www.rcgp.org.uk/pdf/ISS_SUMM02_13.pdf

Foundation Programme website
www.foundationprogramme.nhs.uk/

Tooke Report
www.mmcinquiry.org.uk/draft.htm

MMC and the Gold Guide
www.mmc.nhs.uk

Chapter 11 What is it like to be a Physician?

Amit Bali

Picture the scene: you are at a social gathering. You meet a person for the first time and when asked what it is you do for a living (the traditional, yet unimaginative ice-breaker) you answer that you are a physician. The reflex reply is invariably: 'What do you specialise in?' To those outside the world of medicine, the term 'general medicine' tends to provoke quizzical looks and shrugging of shoulders. The Royal College of Physicians commissioned a survey on this very topic in 2007. There was definite confusion as to the definition of the term 'physician'; in fact, 37 per cent of people questioned actually thought that physicians were surgeons! Perhaps in keeping with the popular view of doctors as specialists, the Royal College defines physicians as 'specialists in the diagnosis and treatment of medical conditions'. To the uninitiated, however, this probably does not provide any further clarity. In fact, it is easier to describe everything a physician is not: no operations, no children and no women's bits. Everything else in hospital medicine comes under the umbrella of the physician.

What does being a Physician involve?

In essence, general medicine is what it says on the tin, and therein lies the challenge – the humble physician must be all things to all people. So, what's it like to actually do the job? This is probably best looked at by examining the many different duties that a physician has, and by looking at a typical week's work. A senior physician has to deal with the acute and the chronic, the inpatient and the outpatient – and, more importantly, be able to switch between the roles without missing a beat. The duties themselves may vary depending on the exact sub-specialty of medicine they may have chosen, but there are certainly some roles that most trainee physicians will have to fulfil. For example, the on-call senior physician (a duty that will be performed at least once a week and which is possibly the busiest job in the hospital) is responsible for every new patient who needs to stay in hospital and does not fit into the above 'other' categories. They are also the 'go-to-guy' for every other team in the hospital (and, indeed, every general practitioner in the local area). A general surgeon with a patient who has just come out of the operating theatre who has trouble breathing, or an 'orthopod' who has fixed a frail lady's hip only to find that she now has a crushing chest pain will both call the medical Registrar then breathe a sigh of relief when the phone is placed down and the buck is firmly passed. However, this should not put off budding doctors – in fact, such a role is aspired to by many, and admired by all others. Such responsibility is earned through years of training, with knowledge cumulatively accrued like reward points on a supermarket loyalty card (but used far more regularly). A doctor in this position will have spent many years gaining experience and earning their stripes in a junior role before he or she is let loose. Even then, of course, a physician does not work alone, and there will always be team of colleagues performing these tasks as a group.

The one thing that general medicine is not is boring – in fact it has the greatest variety of all areas of medicine – and there are other components in the day of a physician. Once a medical team has admitted a patient into their care, they must do exactly that: look after them. This again involves a team of varying ranks, from the Consultant (not these days preceded by the words 'god-like') to the house officer (now called a Foundation Year 1 doctor). Typically around 30 patients with a wide range of medical problems will be under the watch of each team. Each day they do a ward round to chart each patient's progress, make a plan and carry it out. This is where the caricature of professorial physicians as beard-stroking intellectuals is at its most obvious. Each patient is examined regularly, any tests or investigations analysed and appropriate changes to their management made. These can include changes in medications, a clinical procedure or more investigations to aid management of the disease process. In addition to this, a physician must also consider other, non-medical ways in which the patient's condition can be improved. For example, a patient whose heart failure is improving may need physiotherapy to improve their mobility, social support to obtain suitable housing and occupational therapy assessment to discover their ability to function with their usual daily activities. Each ward round therefore creates a long set of 'jobs' for the junior doctors, who must roam around the hospital completing them.

Junior doctors on the team will usually spend the majority of their time on their respective wards. As well as performing the tasks from the ward round, they will be contacted regarding any new developments for their patients during the day. This could include the results of blood tests and scans, arranging referrals to other specialties or planning for the patient's discharge into the community, with constant reminders from the nursing staff via regular bleeps (a necessary yet often annoying feature of the day). In all honesty, many of these tasks can leave junior doctors feeling like administration staff, but the role is vital to ensure that the team functions well, and that the patients get the best possible care. Equally, it means that the junior doctors will have in-depth knowledge of their patients, develop deeper relationships with them and hence are viewed by the patients and their families as their first point of contact. It is therefore common to have to counsel patients on their condition, which encompasses giving them information, discussing treatment options and sometimes breaking bad news. Nobody can deny the importance of such a relationship; the rapport between doctor and patient at its best.

In the meantime, during the day, senior physicians often have outpatient clinics. Here, plans are made for patients with chronic, long-standing conditions which require monitoring. General practitioners across the area will also refer new patients for the physician's expert opinion. These should be patients well enough to be at home, but who require regular input on the management of their condition(s). There are opportunities for junior doctors to be introduced to the world of outpatients, learning from the senior physician's consultation style, their manner and their clinical decision-making.

The general nature of a physician's working life is, for many, its attraction. It is difficult to get bored when each bleep is unpredictable, each referral letter different. However, those looking for something more specialised can do just that – general medicine can be split up via the different systems of the body, to give heart specialists, lung specialists and so on. In fact, the Royal College of Physicians lists 26 sub-specialties, from allergy medicine to stroke medicine. This offers yet another variation, namely the opportunity to delve deep into one of these areas and become an eminent expert in a chosen sub-specialty. You can do this without losing the general aspect too – a gastroenterologist, for example, will normally be expected to fulfil general on-call duties. An added attraction for many to go down the specialist route is the opportunity to perform highly specialised procedures such as angioplasties and colonoscopies.

Don't worry if all of this sounds more than a bit daunting. There is a strong culture of teaching in general medicine – perhaps more so than any other specialty – so that every person's knowledge and experience rubs off on their colleagues. Equally, a physician will never be working on their own; they work in teams, so there is always a level of support, a second opinion or someone to bounce ideas off. A physician will get to know their colleagues closely (especially those on the same team), with the similar interests and shared experiences usually leading to lasting friendships. It is this, in combination with the variety and rewarding nature of the work, that makes general medicine so fascinating. The opportunity to have a job so interesting, so rich in terms of the experiences gained, and to play such an important role in the lives of so many, is indeed a great privilege.

What qualities should a Physician possess?

The qualities needed to be a good physician reflect the nature of the patients seen – that is, a wide variety of virtues. The extremely sick patient attending accident and emergency requires a sharp-witted, highly intelligent and, above all, decisive doctor that can cope under immense pressures, applying a library's worth of knowledge at will. The patient requiring a high-risk emergency procedure will equally require a doctor with a steady hand and nerves of steel.

Away from the emergency setting, a physician on the medical ward will need to be organised, systematic and methodical, as a list of over 30 patients is usual. These will range from the sick to the social (i.e. may have been unwell, but now need improved housing or physiotherapy before they can be discharged). That brings us on to communication, a quality required by all physicians. There has been a realisation within the profession in recent years that doctors need training to polish their communication skills; serious medical conditions obviously have massive repercussions for the patients affected by them, so a physician must be empathetic, understanding and a good listener.

By their nature, a physician will be inquisitive, and want to keep up-to-date with the latest trends and treatments in medicine. The 'evidence-based medicine' approach has grown as the profession has realised the importance of improving practice, but with a balanced, objective attitude to research and auditing current practices. Striving to better oneself and hence be the best possible doctor is what underpins general medicine's reputation, both within the profession and amongst the general public.

How do you become a Physician?

Decision making time comes during your foundation years (see Chapter 10). Currently, budding physicians must apply for two years of Core Medical Training (part of Specialty Training), which is designed to give a core background in general internal medicine. A prospective applicant should look to expand their CV in preparation for this, with relevant examples of management experience, communication skills, and involvement in teaching and research. If selected for interview candidates undergo a standardised interview process, often encompassing clinical scenarios, a brief presentation and, of course, the obligatory 'why do you want to do medicine?' All the world's a stage, and courses exist to enable trainee doctors to polish their performance. In a year or two a written examination is likely to be added to the selection process, testing applicants' decision making skills and aptitude.

At present, this process must be repeated after these two years, and doctors must re-apply to sub-specialties. As the positions increase in seniority, so does the requirement of courses and post-graduate qualifications.

Professional exams

To progress to become a fully qualified physician and advance along the Specialty Training pathway, a doctor must obtain the necessary postgraduate qualification. The Royal College of Physicians is the body which oversees this, with their membership examination, the MRCP. These consist of three parts: MRCP Part I, which assesses basic science knowledge; Part II written which tests your clinical acumen; and Part II clinical (also called PACES) which assesses practical clinical skills and interpretation. These examinations are tough, but few would doubt that they are a necessary step to ensure adequate training and that senior doctors have reached an acceptable standard.

Options within Medicine

Although the appeal for some is the chance to become a 'generalist', for many the opportunity to specialise allows them to focus further on areas they have enjoyed during their training. As previously mentioned, the Royal College of Physicians has identified 26 such sub-specialties. They are: Acute Medicine, Allergy, Audiological Medicine, Cardiology, Clinical Genetics, Clinical Neurophysiology, Clinical Pharmacology and Therapeutics, Dermatology, Endocrinology and Diabetes Mellitus, Gastroenterology, General (Internal) Medicine, Genitourinary Medicine, Geriatric Medicine, Haematology, Immunology,

Infectious Diseases, Medical Oncology, Medical Ophthalmology, Metabolic Medicine, Neurology, Nuclear Medicine, Paediatric Cardiology, Palliative Medicine, Pharmaceutical Medicine, Rehabilitation Medicine, Renal Medicine, Respiratory Medicine, Rheumatology, Sport and Exercise Medicine, and Stroke Medicine. Additionally, there are options to broaden horizons outside of direct clinical care. Many hospitals around the country are teaching hospitals, where physicians can get involved with schooling the next generation of doctors. As previously mentioned, research is of utmost importance to the profession as a whole and hence to patient care. The world of academic medicine also includes this aspect, with the chance for physicians to become directly involved with innovative and ground-breaking research.

Summary

As the opportunities within general medicine are seemingly endless, the aim of this chapter is to offer the merest glimpse into the available avenues, whilst emphasising the broad, wide-ranging foundation upon which these options are built. Although difficult to define, life as a physician remains the most varied, diverse and, therefore, challenging specialty within medicine. This assortment of options suits a large number of training doctors who are not exactly sure in which direction they wish their career to proceed. Usually, this is because their interests spread across a variety of disciplines, and the decision of which areas of interest to discard is a tough one. General medicine is unique in allowing someone in this position to further their knowledge, skills and experience in multiple fields, all the while keeping the option of specialising open. Along the way, a physician becomes a more shrewd, skilled, smart doctor (a personal source of pride to anyone who achieves it) and, more importantly, the doctor every patient wants to treat them.

Key points:

- Would appeal to those looking for a varied, challenging, yet rewarding career in medicine

- Ranges from emergency, life-threatening situations to the management of chronic disease

- Teamwork, both with other doctors and other disciplines, is paramount

- Exams to be passed along the way, but relevant to everyday practice

- Still retain the option to sub-specialise later.

Chapter 12 Life as a Surgeon – What is all the hype?

Chris Thompson

Being a surgeon is great fun. That's the reason why most surgeons are surgeons. It is really quite fascinating to see what goes on inside our bodies and it's the surgeon's great privilege to witness nature's complexity and beauty first hand, both with the eyes and the fingertips.

A surgical day usually begins early (before 8am) with a ward round. This is when the surgeon makes time to see the patients under their care in the hospital wards. These patients may be people who have come in for, or are recovering from, a planned operation, or people who have come in as an acute emergency either via the GP or the Emergency Department. Decisions are made about the investigation or management of each patient and the Surgeon's junior doctors busy themselves carrying out these instructions for the next few hours.

Surgeons do not only work in the hospital wards and operating theatres; they also work in clinics seeing patients who have been referred from GPs and following up their own post-operative patients. They also spend time helping with the management of the hospital at large. Increasingly, more complex cases, particularly those involving cancer, are discussed by surgeons at multidisciplinary meetings with many different doctors and allied health professionals lending their expertise to patient management.

Obviously, a considerable proportion of a surgeon's time is

spent performing operations in the operating theatre. Apart from operations themselves, a great deal of teaching and learning takes place. Surgical trainees get practical experience under supervision and are talked through the more simple procedures. The great thing about operations is that, just like people, every operation is different. The benefit of long experience can be telling, particularly when unforeseen emergencies take place. In fact the best surgeons never seem to have emergency situations because they are so calm under pressure when unexpected things happen or, more commonly, they have foreseen the danger and prevented it from ever occurring.

A day in the life of a surgical trainee

'*My working day officially starts at 8am and finishes at 5pm, but in reality the day is as long as it needs to be to complete the work and may stray outside these hours. During this time my responsibilities include looking after the inpatients, attending clinic and helping with the operating lists.*

From time to time I am "on-call". This means that I see all the new people admitted into the hospital as an emergency. I assess them and start off the management of their problem. This is a 12 hour shift and can be either at night or during the day. I am on a rota with seven other doctors, meaning that I am on-call one day in six (one person is on nights you see) and on nights one week in seven (for seven nights). I find these on-call shifts to be great fun. The pressure of trying to keep up with what is going on is really stimulating. I also feel that if the on-call job is done well the new patients can really benefit.

There are some obvious negatives to my job. The hours are long (but getting better and certainly better than they once were), which curtails the hobbies you can pursue outside of work. My brother is a dentist, and works from nine until five. When we shared a house together he would regularly say that he never saw me because of the hours I worked. The other big drawback is that it is very difficult to say where you will be working from year to year. That means that it is difficult to set down roots and call somewhere "home", which becomes increasingly important as you get older. The work happens in a high pressure environment – let's face it, when you have promised someone that you will make them better with an operation, the pressure is truly on. There is out of hours work that has to be done, and believe me it is difficult to work a long week and be motivated enough to revise for an exam whilst trying to have a life outside work. But anyone who thinks it can't be done is wrong.'

What qualities should a Surgeon possess?

Surgeons should possess the same qualities that all good doctors possess, and maybe a couple more.

- A logical and enquiring mind.
- A thoughtful and caring approach to communication with patients, their relatives and work colleagues.
- Calmness under pressure allowing the mind and body to work swiftly together.
- A flair for leadership and management.
- The ability to cope with change both within the medical sphere and in the wider context of healthcare delivery.
- Dexterity (for some this is natural but it can be learned to some extent too).
- A lifelong approach to learning both from the published literature and from experiences gained within clinical practice – this helps to keep the surgeon abreast of the latest developments in the field so they can deliver these benefits to the patients as they occur.

Overall, a surgeon is a caring and well informed doctor, who has the extra skill of being able to perform operations. A surgeon is not simply a mechanic of the body.

How do you become a Surgeon?

To become a surgeon is a big undertaking, which means dedicating a great proportion of your life to learning and training.

The first step is to be offered a place at medical school and gain the necessary grades to be able to accept it. Medical school itself is great fun but very hard work. Many medical students with an interest in surgery join in with their local surgical society and participate in surgically related workshops and lectures. For anyone considering surgery as a career, this type of extra-curricular activity can really help to give you a competitive advantage when it comes to job applications.

Once you have completed medical school, training to be a surgeon truly begins.

Training

Surgical careers and surgical training are currently in a state of flux, as is the rest of medical training (see Chapter 10). This is because of the European Working Time Directive and Modernising Medical Careers. In reality it is very hard to say how surgical careers will be structured in years to come, so the current system will be described as a model.

All medical training is attempting to move towards a system of 'competency acquisition' rather than a simple experiential, apprenticeship style of learning. A competency could be loosely described as the ability to do something independently in a safe and effective manner. The new training system uses a continuous assessment system of workplace-based assessments, appraisals and academic examinations to monitor a trainee surgeon's progress towards becoming a consultant. Training doesn't end when you become a consultant though; there are advances being made all the time, so even when training is complete a continuous 'life-long learning' approach is required. In fact it is the rapid manner in which change occurs that makes all of medicine so interesting and rewarding.

The career path for a surgical trainee after graduation from medical school has three parts.

Foundation Years 1 and 2. These are years in which the trainee learns the basic skills required to work as a doctor in any field of medicine.

Core Surgical Training Years 1 and 2. These are the junior years of specialty training. Trainees build on their basic skills and experience from the Foundation Years and take exams to become a member of the Royal College of Surgery. Oddly, this means that the trainee's title returns from Doctor to Mister or Miss – a throwback to the days when surgeons were part of the Guild of Barbers!

Specialty Training. This is the final stage before completion of training. During this time the trainee takes on more responsibility and becomes more and more independent in their practise. An 'exit' exam is taken (see below). The trainee develops his or her own specialist interest within their chosen specialty and often undertakes some clinical research. This stage can vary in its length but generally takes six to ten years.

It is planned that either during the foundation or core years of training a trainee will decide which of the nine surgical specialties he or she wishes to work in. As the trainee becomes more senior, the training received will become increasingly focussed towards this chosen specialty.

There is a competitive interviewing process for entry into Core Surgical Training and Specialty Training. There will be further competition to join the specialty desired and even stiffer competition for consultant jobs. The truth is that the whole process is competitive and if that doesn't suit you, surgery may not be the right career for you.

Similar to UCAS for universities, the process for entering surgical training involves an application form and an interview. There aren't enough jobs for all the applicants in just the same way that there are more applicants for medical school than there are places, so it is important to put yourself at the head of the pack to give yourself the best chance to succeed.

On the application form the candidate has to show that they have made reasonable attempts to experience surgery and have developed a keen interest in it. To tick enough boxes to get an interview most need to have had some surgical experience during the foundation years, participated in audits or research work with a surgical slant, and attended courses of a surgical nature such as Basic Surgical Skills or Advanced Trauma Life Support. Interviewing in itself is an art form and the author does not pretend to know any sure-fire answers to get you through. One piece of useful advice is that being yourself and letting your personality show certainly improves your chances of success. If you really do want it and are committed, it will shine through on the day.

Professional exams
During surgical training there are two major exams.

Firstly, the Membership of The Royal College of Surgeons

(MRCS) exam. This is a two part exam, taken during the Core Training period.

Part A is a four hour multiple-choice examination which tests knowledge of the applied sciences of medicine and clinical problem solving. A comprehensive knowledge of anatomy, physiology and pathology and their application in the real world is needed.

Part B is an Objective Structured Clinical Examination (OSCE). This may well be a new concept to you now, but one with which you will become very familiar as you progress through your training. The exam consists of stations (16 in all) where the candidate has the opportunity to demonstrate their competence as a surgeon. These stations may require them to answer questions in an interview style (known as viva voce), role play (to test communication), examine a patient, take a history or demonstrate their dexterity and spatial awareness. This gruelling process takes around three hours and is a true test of mental stamina as well as knowledge.

Once these two exams are passed the candidate may change his or her title back to Mr or Miss, as previously described.

Towards the end of specialty training an exit exam, the FRCS (Fellowship of the Royal College of Surgeons), is taken. This exam comes in three parts: a written, oral and clinical part. Following this exam the candidate is able to 'exit' from training and enter the wider world of consultant grade positions.

Options within surgery

Surgery covers nine specialties; the careers that they offer are vastly different from one another and range from life and death emergency work to intricately planned surgery bordering on art. The specialties are:

- General surgery – all things abdominal, breast and vascular (blood vessels)
- Orthopaedics – bones
- Neurosurgery – brains
- Plastics – not just boobs and tummy tucks! But also burns and reconstruction following severe, disfiguring injury
- Urology – the waterworks
- Ear nose and throat – self explanatory
- Paediatrics – child surgery
- Maxillofacial – the super dentists
- Cardiothoracic – hearts and lungs.

These nine specialties are further subdivided into smaller sub-specialties. This division of divisions helps to provide patients with increasingly more expert practitioners, which means that better care can be delivered. For example, general surgery can be broken down into breast surgery, colorectal (the large bowel, rectum and anus) surgery, upper gastrointestinal surgery, hepatobilliary (liver and gall bladder) surgery and vascular surgery. All these subspecialties have their own set of operations in which the surgeons specialise.

Summary
Surgery is a fulfilling and varied career which not only provides stimulating and exciting work for the Surgeon, but also, and most importantly, does a great deal of good for people of all ages and backgrounds. In the words of a surgical trainee:

> 'All in I find my job to be interesting and varied with multiple differing challenges, both mental and physical. There aren't

many jobs that stay as interesting as mine has, which is probably the reason why I like it so much.'

Key points:

- The life of a surgeon is varied and involves much more than just operating

- Surgery is very popular and you need to show determination to succeed in this field

- Training to be a surgeon takes at least ten years in most cases

- Once trained as a surgeon you can specialise in lots of different things

Chapter 13 Psychiatry – what's it all about?

Jamie Wilson

Psychiatry is the medical specialty that often arouses most curiosity in prospective doctors. Its reputation, after all, is laden with cultural myths. With its long heritage of colourful characters such as Freud, and coverage in the media and other cultural domains, preconceptions can fuel attitudes to it as a potential career path. While such views are still evident in society as a whole, they also continue in mainstream medicine. This can skew what advice or perspective you gain of psychiatry during medical school. Limited experience of dealing with mental illness and psychological distress means that many doctors are not skilled in dealing with the nuances of mental health problems.

Psychiatry in its most literal form is the study of the mind. However, much of the work of general psychiatrists deals with the assessment, treatment and long term management of individuals with what are termed 'severe and enduring' mental illnesses such as schizophrenia and bipolar disorder (previously known as manic depression). In the UK, to become a psychiatrist you must have been to medical school and completed your foundation year training. After this period, you are in a position to choose a specialty. It can seem a long time to wait before embarking on a specialty that is fundamentally different from other medical specialties. Why, you might ask, do I not train as a psychologist if I want to learn about the mind and deal with patients with psychological difficulties?

This is valid question that you should ponder before you consider applying to medical school. It took me seven years from the start of medical school to start my psychiatric training. Could that time not have been better spent? The answer to this is that you are in a unique position if you have medical training behind you. It is then possible to integrate an understanding of psychology, psychotherapy and some of the other intellectual disciplines of psychiatry into the framework you have established over the preceding years.

Medical training allows you to come at psychiatry from the perspective of a doctor whose aim is to diagnose and treat a patient. I think many psychiatrists would agree with me that mental health problems are given some validity within a medical diagnostic model. Thinking of mental health problems as medical conditions does not underestimate the complex nature of mental health problems which often arise from a blend of biological, social and psychological sources. However, being under the care of a doctor can help a patient recover from being 'ill', whether that be due a form of depression, psychosis or other disorder such as anorexia nervosa where physical and mental aspects are entwined. I've just tried to simplify this a bit for readers who might be new to this idea.

Mental health services in the UK are an example of where the multidisciplinary model of care is most embedded. The traditional hierarchy of medicine is replaced by a flat team of psychiatrists, psychologists, social workers, occupational therapists and mental health nurses. It can often be a cultural shock to transfer to this kind of setting from a more typical medical specialty. Nonetheless, psychiatrists are in a position to wed together the different viewpoints and perspectives of team members and patients. As a doctor, it is likely you will already have dealt with some exceptionally stressful circumstances in your training. Many of the multidisciplinary colleagues you encounter in psychiatry will not have had the exposure to the gruelling shifts and training you have been through. This means that you will generally be able to digest and act upon fluid situations more quickly than other team members through the experience you have gained.

What exactly does a Psychiatrist do?

As a trainee psychiatrist, you will normally be allocated to the care of a consultant, in the first two years either in general adult or old age psychiatry. Often this will be in a community mental health team (CMHT), which will have several hundred patients under its care for a specific postcode. You may be required to work between this community setting and an in-patient ward where patients have often been detained under the Mental Health Act.

Typically your week will consist of outpatient clinics, ward rounds, home visits and teaching. Psychiatry has a strong reputation for education and you can often expect between three and eight hours of teaching hours each week, with case presentations, psychotherapy supervision, journal clubs, and an allocated hour with your consultant to discuss pastoral issues and difficult cases.

During outpatient clinics, you will assess referrals, conducting a comprehensive psychiatric history that lasts up to 90 minutes. Many of the other patients will be long standing and require reviews of their medication, mental state, risk, general medical issues, housing, and other social factors. Ward rounds are considerably longer than those found in medical specialties. Other time available is spent dictating discharge summaries, which provide a detailed account of a patient's inpatient stay, and other duties such as liaising with relatives and organising referrals to other medical specialties and services within mental health.

Depending on your rota, you may do an evening or night shift once a week or fortnight. This can involve any range of tasks, including assessing patients in A&E, dealing with ward emergencies, and administrative tasks such as writing up drug charts and prescriptions.

Later on in your training, you will spend some time in other specialties such as substance misuse, forensic psychiatry and psychotherapy.

What does being a Psychiatrist involve?

Many people query the distinction between a psychiatrist, psychologist and psychotherapist. Psychotherapy is a talking therapy practised according to an underlying theory that usually involves a therapist and patient, although can sometimes take place with couples, families, and in groups.

The different roles these professionals take on can be confusing. It is best to think of a psychiatrist as a medical doctor who treats mental illness. Thus psychiatrists are able to prescribe psychiatric medication and manage physical health problems, while also acquiring psychotherapy skills and an understanding of psychological issues. Generally, the consultant psychiatrist will lead the team and delegate responsibilities, manage resources, and plan service provision, while keeping a caseload of more complex patients and supervising trainees. A psychologist has completed a doctorate in clinical psychology, and has gained skills usually in psychometric testing (such as IQ), and various forms of psychotherapy such as cognitive behavioural therapy. Psychologists are not able to prescribe medication, and are rarely able to use the Mental Health Act, although this is in the process of changing at the time of writing.

Psychiatrists can also train in psychotherapy. There is increasing emphasis on this, although psychologists are more experienced and do most of the assessment and referrals for psychotherapy. Psychotherapists are usually trained in one particular modality of psychotherapy, such as psychodynamic therapy. Psychotherapists often practice independently in the private sector and work part time in the NHS in some instances.

What qualities should a Psychiatrist possess?

Many of the attributes that will allow you to become a competent psychiatrist are different to those found in mainstream medicine. Some may argue these qualities are not as well defined and are a bit 'woolly' or 'soft'. I would argue they are good life skills that will stand you in good stead in whatever you do, as they will allow you to be flexible and stress-tolerant. Any career in medicine is demanding and you need to ensure that you are at your best, even in times of adversity. As you mature into your late twenties and thirties, other demands become increasingly prominent with family and financial commitments as well as the requirements of your daily career. This list is not exhaustive, but details some of my thoughts on what will help you.

Tolerance of uncertainty

There is considerable emphasis on managing risk in modern psychiatry. This is partly due to political pressure to prevent 'mad' people doing unpredictable things. High profile cases of murders by the mentally ill have exacerbated this problem. Unfortunately, severe forms of psychosis can occasionally result in this outcome, which is evidently devastating for a victim and their relatives. But it is unlikely you will encounter many cases of seriously high risk patients in terms of their risk to others unless you choose a career in forensic psychiatry. It is far more likely that your patients may threaten to harm themselves. This can be extremely stressful if you have had little prior exposure to this kind of scenario. You can feel the weight of responsibility on your shoulders, yet at the same time recognise that it is impossible to entirely eliminate the risk. This aspect of psychiatry is perhaps the most significant in determining how trainees adapt to the pressures. It can be very much down to your underlying temperament. Overall, I did not have many sleepless nights when I was training, but I would be being dishonest if I did not admit that some patients left me feeling worried about what they would do. If you are someone who needs iron cast certainty in your life, psychiatry may not be for you.

Persuasiveness

You may think this is what politicians or advertising executives are good at. But, spending time trying to understand and talk things over with patients, their relatives, and staff members will get you a long way. One of the unique aspects of psychiatry is you are placed in a powerful position of being able to detain people under the Mental Health Act. This is a considerable responsibility and can understandably be perceived by patients, and many other parties, as unnecessary or coercive. You may experience hostility or disbelief and will often encounter patients whose insight into their difficulties is impaired by their disturbed psychological functioning. Even in these circumstances, and perhaps more so, you need to spend time outlining your views and explaining clearly and calmly to those who need to hear. When I say that persuasiveness is an important attribute, I do not mean that you should over-elaborate or minimise certain issues; I merely refer to utilising all your empathic resources and being able to articulate a resonant and compelling viewpoint. This will alleviate some of the anxiety felt by your patients and bolster the strength of the therapeutic relationship, which is vital to their recovery and health.

Delaying gratification

Are you someone who needs instant results? If so, psychiatry may not be your calling. I suggest you go and do surgery, or perhaps working on the trading floor as a broker would suit you better. It is rare that you can 'cure' a patient with mental illness. In fact, it is a bit of myth that you can cure most people with any form of physical or mental illness. Many infectious diseases have been eradicated by immunisation and with an ageing population the burden of chronic disease increases every decade. In psychiatry people suffering from disorders such as depression can take many months to show signs of recovery. You are unlikely to witness immediate results from any intervention you undertake. But a more pleasing aspect is that it can be your skill and expertise that has an impact on recovery more so than drugs and other physical treatments. By acting as a constant presence through a difficult and painful episode in someone's life, you may be able to alter someone's outlook or psychological functioning for the better, thus turning a crisis into an opportunity. This can be very rewarding, but requires patience not expediency. You should also not underestimate the access to an individual's innermost thoughts and feelings you are privy to. I have met some exceptionally interesting patients and the time you are afforded – far more than in other specialties – allows you to form strong bonds with your patients, and is an opportunity that few people, even other doctors, experience.

Support for the underdog

Medicine still retains a glamorous aura for those who seek to pursue it as a career. Do not be fooled. While some specialties offer a more enthralling ride, I know very few doctors who think the glamour matches the TV soaps or cut and thrust of programmes such as ER. Medicine is incredibly hard work and you will often find yourselves dealing with the most downtrodden and vulnerable people in society. Nowhere is this more common than in psychiatry. It is true that mental illness can affect anyone, but you should be under no illusions that the mentally ill often occupy the most deprived and destitute areas of our inner cities. They are often voiceless and neglected by the political agenda. This is particularly so in urban areas where drugs and alcohol misuse can complicate the picture. While funding has improved in some areas in recent years, resources are still lacking in many regions.

Your patience can be tested to the limit when you face barriers concerning discrimination, housing and finding employment. Bureaucracy and internal battles with management around finding a bed or adequate nursing levels add to the frustration. Do you enjoy standing up for people? I happen to believe such an outlook can be helpful. For instance, I get a kick out of challenging people who make prejudicial comments about mental illness on the basis of spurious evidence or ignorance (you would be amazed at how common this happens with other doctors). A fighting spirit, a liberal attitude, and a willingness to look at things differently will place you in a strong position and make the job more rewarding.

How do you become a Psychiatrist?

After five or six years at medical school you are required to do two foundation years which may include a rotation in psychiatry. At the time of writing, specialty training for psychiatry lasts six years until you reach the point where a certificate of the completion of training (CCT) is issued (see Chapter 10).

During medical school, you may wish to consider doing an intercalated BSc. in psychology, neuroscience or a social science to improve your CV and gain some understanding of these areas. Psychiatry placements at medical school are generally brief and last no more than eight weeks. It can be difficult to form an impression during this time, especially if you are not inspired by your placement.

If you have some inkling you would like to pursue psychiatry as a career, you should try and seek out opportunities in areas such as special study modules, research and voluntary work to augment the experience you have gained elsewhere. There is lots of additional information on the Royal College of Psychiatrists website www.rcpsych.ac.uk

Professional exams?

Membership of the Royal College of Psychiatrists is the professional qualification that acts as a gateway to practising independently as a psychiatrist. The exam is now split into three stages with the first two exams taking the form of multiple choice questions on various subjects such as neuroscience, psychology, and other basic sciences as well as the psychiatric sub-specialties. The final exam is a practical exercise similar in format to an objective structured clinical examination (OSCE) that medical students take. These exams are supplemented by workplace based assessments that are conducted while on the training rotation and comprise discrete assessment of core skills such as mental state examination, cognitive examination and risk assessment.

Options within psychiatry

General adult psychiatry
This sub-specialty deals with the majority of referrals and cases in psychiatry. A typical case load will include patients with schizophrenia, bipolar disorder, depression, anxiety disorders such as obsessive compulsive disorder, and many more cases that do not require referral on to further sub-specialties.

Old age psychiatry
Dealing with people over the age 65, much of the case load is patients with dementia such as Alzheimer's and other neuro-degenerative disorders. Patients who have long standing mental illnesses such as schizophrenia who are in this age bracket are also managed by old age psychiatrists.

Crisis teams/Home treatment
A new specialty, these teams attempt to treat patients who are on the cusp of requiring hospital admission with intensive home support by administering medication and managing risk.

Assertive outreach
This service is for particularly severe cases where lesser community treatment has proved ineffective. Many of the patients under the care of these teams require 'depot' medication (long-lasting drugs given by injection) and intensive monitoring.

Liaison psychiatry
This sub-specialty exists at the interface of physical and mental health. Liaison psychiatrists are often requested to assess patients on medical wards to assess capacity to consent to operations and other procedures. Work is varied and

stimulating. If you miss mainstream medicine, this may be the psychiatric sub-specialty to suit your interests.

Substance misuse
Alcohol and other substance misuse such as opiates, amphetamines and cannabis is common in the UK. Specialist services exist to facilitate detoxification and encourage abstinence for individuals who develop dependence to these substances.

Forensic psychiatry
This is a competitive sub-specialty that deals with mentally disturbed offenders. Much of the work is done in prisons or secure hospitals such as Broadmoor. There is considerable scope for court work and an interface with an understanding of law.

Child and adolescent psychiatry
These services provide for children and teenagers with mental health problems as well as spending considerable time working with their families. There is a strong orientation towards psychotherapy in the form of family therapy.

Eating disorders
Anorexia nervosa and bulimia nervosa are the most well recognised eating disorders. Anorexia is among the most serious mental illnesses and can be difficult to treat effectively. Often, inpatient admission is required along with monitoring of nutritional and physical state. A strong focus on psychological work also exists in this specialty.

Psychotherapy
Although some psychiatrists choose to specialise in psychotherapy, this is a relatively small subspecialty. Doctors generally

train in psychodynamic psychotherapy, which is a form of talking therapy that draws on unconscious processes, early life experiences and the relationship between the therapist and patient to explain their current problems.

Summary

Psychiatry is a broad and stimulating specialty that will open your eyes to an array of social and anthropological issues. Every patient seems unique, which is not always the case in mainstream medicine where the focus is on disease and pathology rather than the holistic focus in psychiatry. Progress in neuroscience as well as exposure to more traditional modalities such as psychotherapy make for an interesting blend of learning, and you will be well supported in your professional development and educational needs. You will also be responsible for dealing with some of society's most vulnerable people, which makes for a challenging yet rewarding career.

Key points:

- Psychiatrists deal with the assessment, treatment and management of mental illness

- Psychiatrists work very closely with other health professionals such as social workers and psychologists

- To be a psychiatrist it helps to be tolerant, patient and persuasive

- You can choose to specialize in a wide range of things including psychotherapy, forensics and substance misuse